SECOND EDITION

Ethical Dilemmas

IN LONG-TERM CARE

Study Edition

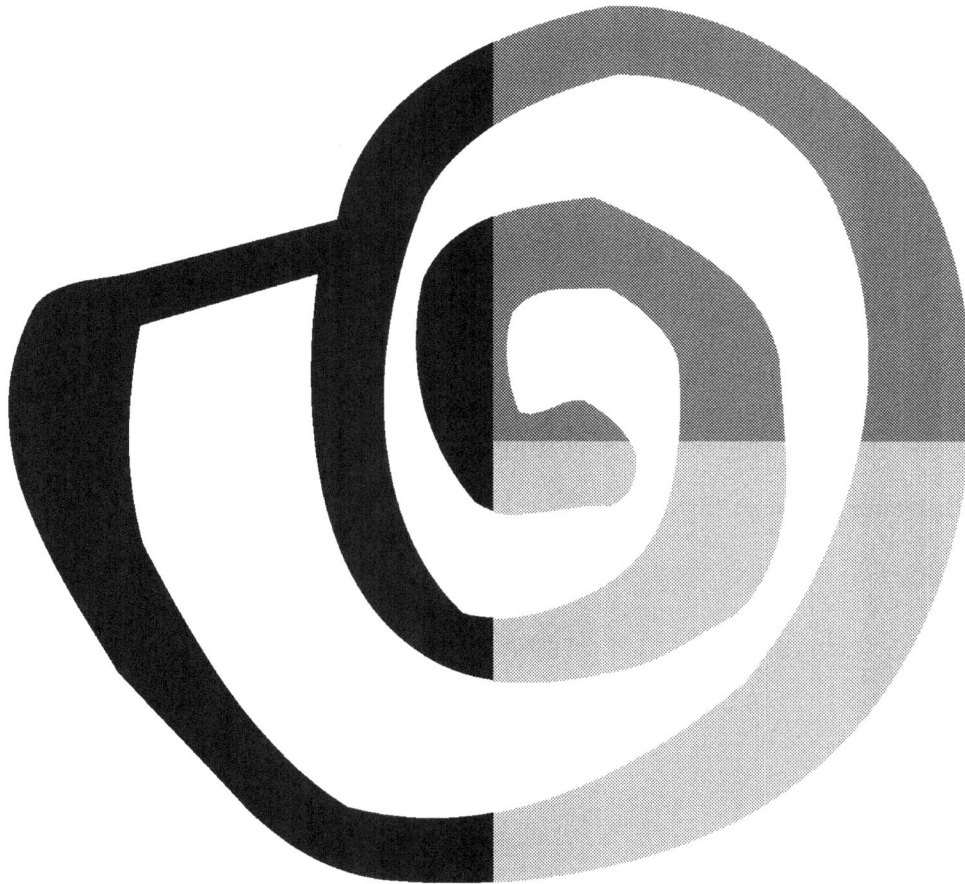

Janine M. Idziak
Loras College

NOTICE AND DISCLAIMER

Cover and book design and layout: Imaging Design Studio, Kelly J. Fassbinder

Facilitator's Edition ISBN: 978-1-58254-023-8

Study Edition ISBN: 978-1-58254-024-5

Printed in the United States of America

With gratitude to my parents
Jeannette and John Idziak

Contents

Part Four: Special Topics

PREFACE

As evidenced by the development of ethics committees, ethics is increasingly becoming part of the delivery of health care. However, many resources in health care ethics still focus on the acute care setting. Ethical Dilemmas in Long-Term Care, second edition, discusses the standard issues and problems of health care ethics exclusively in the context of case studies in the long-term care setting. It contains as well discussion of ethical issues unique to long-term care in multi-level facilities.

This text provides a comprehensive, in-depth educational program that can be used in modules for staff in-service programs and for educating members of ethics committees. It has been prepared in two editions: a *Study Edition* and a *Facilitator's Edition*.

The study edition contains topical chapters, each of which has the same structure. The introductory section lists the issues to be considered in the chapter. The chapter includes one or more case studies describing concrete situations in which these issues arise, with expository sections discussing the issues. At the end of the chapter is a section entitled "For Group Discussion." This section invites readers to become active participants in doing ethics. It provides the opportunity to think through the material in the chapter and to apply the principles presented. A listing of resources appropriate for further study of the topic is given at the end of the chapter.

The Facilitator's Edition contains all the topical chapters plus a listing of audio-visual and Internet resources for each topic. The case studies used in the chapters and the "For Group Discussion" sections are excerpted on a worksheet that can be reproduced for educational purposes. This edition also contains an analysis of the case studies presented in "For Group Discussion."

The case studies included in this book are hypothetical but are based on particular cases or types of cases that have occurred. The hypothetical nature of the cases is intended to preserve confidentiality. The case studies are written as if they are currently going on. This has been done deliberately to simulate the actual ethical decision-making process. When we have to make a tough ethical decision, we often do not know exactly what outcome will occur. This is part of the challenge of "doing ethics."

Many books on health care ethics begin with ethical theory and then proceed to apply the various theories and principles to specific dilemmas in health care. However, a pure exposition of ethical theories and principles can seem very abstract and removed from the experience of health care providers, and hence, can prove difficult to understand. For this reason, this book takes a different approach. Ethical principles and theories are introduced in the context of concrete moral dilemmas. At the end of the text, an appendix pulls together in an organized way the various theories and principles presented in the course of the chapters.

Ethical Dilemmas in Long-Term Care can be used for the initial education of ethics committee members when such committees are first formed. Established ethics committees can use this educational program for the orientation of new members, to bring them up to speed with seasoned committee members. Ethics committee members can also use individual chapters for background information when conducting ethics consults.

The Jewish Home and Hospital for the Aged in New York City has received recognition for its pioneering Center on Ethics in Long-Term Care. (1) The Center's educational programming has targeted "professionals from medicine, nursing, social service, administration, dietary, and physical and occupational therapy" as well as paraprofessional staff members such as nursing aides and orderlies. (1) Their project illustrates the wide range of staff members in a long-term care facility who can profit from ethics education. *Ethical Dilemmas in Long-Term Care* can assist other facilities in undertaking a similar project.

Acknowledgments

As a professor of philosophy, my academic work in the field of bioethics has been greatly enriched by the "hands on" experience afforded me by working on and with ethics committees in the long-term care setting. I want to extend my thanks to the Commission on Ethics in Long-Term Care of the American Association of Homes and Services for the Aging in Washington, D.C., to Stonehill Franciscan Services and Bethany Home in Dubuque, Iowa, and to the Dubuque Regional Healthcare Ethics Committee.

My work with the Medical-Moral Commission of the Archdiocese of Dubuque, Iowa in preparing a handbook on health care ethics provided the occasion for extensive searches of the literature on bioethics. These literature searches are reflected in the chapter notes of this book. I am also indebted to Mercy Medical Center in Dubuque for the opportunity to use their library resources in the preparation of this book.

Janine Marie Idziak, Ph.D.
Dubuque, Iowa
June 2002

Note
1. Ellen Olson, Eileen R. Chichin, Leslie S. Libow, Theresa Martico-Greenfield, Richard R. Neufeld, and Michael Mulvihill, "A Center on Ethics in Long-Term Care," The Gerontologist 33/2 (1993): 269-74.

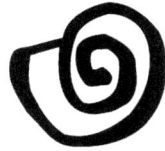

Chapter 1

The Expanding Role of Ethics in Health Care

What Is Ethics?

Ethics asks us to stand back and evaluate our actions. It asks us to judge that some actions ought to be done and that others ought to be avoided.

In the minds of some, ethics consists in nothing but a set of rules governing behavior—rules which have often been superimposed by other people. Ethics is thought of as nothing more than a list of "dos" and "don'ts."

However, contemporary philosophers have presented ethics as an enterprise fostering human happiness and fulfillment. On this view, the purpose of ethical reflection is to consider the choices and courses of action that most promote the fulfillment of persons and the community. (1) Understood in this way, "doing ethics" is a very positive activity.

The Ethical Dimensions of Health Care

Decision making in health care often involves more than just the medical facts of the case. Ethical principles and values will be the determining factor in which course of action is chosen.

Suppose that Betty Smith, aged 81 and a resident of St. Francis Care Center, is terminally ill with pancreatic cancer. At this point in her illness she is experiencing severe pain. The pain is being treated with narcotic medication through the facility's hospice program, but sometimes she has to be sedated to the point of unconsciousness to experience relief. Betty's oncologist estimates that she has only two weeks left to live, at the most. When Betty is awake and lucid, she pleads with the staff to "do something to end her life" so that she can be at peace in heaven with her husband. Betty's children also believe that she should be spared from any further suffering, especially since she is likely to die so soon anyway. On one occasion when they are all visiting their mother, they tell her that they will ask her oncologist to give her an overdose of medication so that she can finally have peace. A licensed practical nurse on the staff overhears this conversation, reports it to the Director of Nursing, who in turn contacts the facility's administrator. The administrator contacts Betty's children and asks them to come in for a special care conference. Betty's children again express the desire for euthanasia for their mother. The administrator firmly tells them that euthanasia cannot be allowed at St. Francis Care Center because its religious tradition unqualifiedly opposes this practice.

Everyone involved likely agrees on the medical facts of this case: Betty is terminally ill with pancreatic cancer, she has at most two weeks to live, and she is experiencing severe pain. However, the administrator of St. Francis Care Center opposes an overdose of medication deliberately being given to Betty because she has a different view of the ethical permissibility of euthanasia than do Betty's children. Not the medical facts of the case but, rather, the respective ethical judgments of the administrator and of Betty's children ultimately determine the course of action they believe ought to be taken.

Many health care facilities now have ethics committees in place (see below). Many large health care systems employ professional ethicists to address ethical issues on a full-time basis. Just as it is common practice to consult with specialists about medical care, so ethics consultation services are now being offered to help patients and residents, families, and health care providers work through difficult ethical dilemmas (see below). The accreditation review of health care facilities by the Joint Commission on Accreditation of Healthcare Organizations (JCAHO) now includes evaluation of a facility's practice of ethics.(2) Ethics has very much become a part of contemporary health care services.

Levels of Ethical Inquiry in Health Care

Ethical issues concerning health care can arise at different levels. Obviously, ethical questions can arise regarding the medical care of individual patients and residents. Should 80-year-old John, who has Alzheimer's disease, be resuscitated if he suffers a cardiac arrest? Should he be given antibiotics if he develops pneumonia? Eleanor has been unconscious for a year, and physicians think it very unlikely that she will ever regain consciousness. Should her tube feeding be discontinued so that she can be allowed to die? These types of questions belong to the category of clinical ethics.

At the same time, ethical questions can arise about how a health care facility or service is operated. For example, ethical questions can be raised about the financing of health care. Is it right for a physician who is part of a health maintenance organization (HMO) to refrain from prescribing a particular drug for an individual who would benefit from it because the drug is too costly? Do long-term care facilities have any obligation to accept as residents individuals who are on Medicaid when the reimbursement level is below the actual cost of care? Ethical questions can also arise regarding a health care facility's treatment of its employees. Was the last merit raise for employees fairly handled? If a health care worker has personal objections in conscience to a course of action being taken for a particular resident (for example, the withdrawal of tube feeding), how should this situation be handled? Can she be forced to participate against her will in a course of action she regards as morally wrong? Yet another concern today is how the ethical value of confidentiality can be preserved with the computerization and electronic transmission of medical records. All of these questions belong to the realm of organizational ethics.

In the context of long-term care, yet another realm of ethical inquiry has been identified. It is described as "everyday ethics":

> On a day-to-day basis, the kinds of issues that the residents of nursing homes confront...are matters that at first glance appear mundane or banal:

Can I eat what I want? Must I have a designated roommate? When can I go out for a walk? Why can't I wake up and go to sleep when I want to? Why can't I wash my clothes in the bathroom sink? What can I wear to dinner? Do I have to take a bath? When can I expect help in using the telephone? Must I sleep with a bed rail up?...

It may seem odd at first even to describe such questions as moral or ethical. But ethics concerns not only questions of life and death but how one ought to live with and interact with others on a daily basis. The ethics of the ordinary is just as much a part of health care ethics as the ethics of the extraordinary. For the resident, the small decisions of daily life set the boundaries of his or her moral universe. (3)

While this book will give primary attention to everyday ethics in the long-term care setting and to issues in clinical ethics, some issues from the realm of organizational ethics will also be addressed.

Ethics Committees: A Resource for Resolving Ethical Dilemmas

Ethics committees have been established at many health care facilities. These committees have a variety of names: medical-moral committee, human values committee, bioethics committee, advisory committee on ethical decision making. (4) While ethics committees began in the acute care, hospital setting, they have expanded to long-term care facilities and other types of health care services.

Ethics committees usually have between twelve and fifteen members. The membership is multidisciplinary, representing various types of work in health care and other professions. The committee is not necessarily made up entirely of employees of the facility; it may include individuals from within the community the facility serves. In a long-term care setting, an ethics committee typically includes representation from the board of trustees, the facility's administrator, the facility's director of nursing and possibly other nursing staff, a physician, area clergy or a representative of the facility's own pastoral care staff, a social worker employed at the facility, an attorney, an ethicist (usually, a philosophy or theology professor), and one or more residents. Many ethics committees serve just one facility. However, a number of facilities in a particular geographical area sometimes join together to establish a regional ethics committee serving all the participating facilities. Some ethics committees meet monthly, others meet bi-monthly, and yet others meet only quarterly.

An ethics committee typically has three functions: education, the development and review of institutional policies and guidelines, and case consultation.

One of the primary functions of an ethics committee is providing education on issues in health care ethics. This includes education of the committee members themselves, who come from a variety of professional backgrounds. It also includes continuing education and in-service programs for the facility's staff. In addition, ethics committees engage in community education, developing programming for the general public. A frequent topic of such community education programs is advance directives.

Second, ethics committees are involved in developing and reviewing policies and guidelines that have an ethical dimension. For example, an ethics committee may develop a policy on artificial nutrition and hydration to be sent to the facility's board of trustees for approval. Or the committee may be asked to review and revise a policy already in place on the use of restraints.

Third, an ethics committee is typically available for consultation with residents, family members, and health care providers about difficult ethical dilemmas they face. Such a meeting with an ethics committee (or sometimes a subcommittee of it) is known as an *ethics consult*.

Residents and family members can discuss the ethical dimensions of treatment decisions with their health care providers, the facility's pastoral care staff, or their own clergy. Health care providers can talk with their co-workers. However, a time may come when residents, family, or health care providers feel that they have reached the limits of their own abilities to address an ethical issue. In such cases an ethics consult may be a helpful resource.

An ethics consult may

- provide information about ethical principles relevant to the case under discussion;

- help clarify what options are open;

- provide information about similar cases;

- provide information about relevant policies of the facility;

- result in recommendations which are *advisory* in nature.

Ethics consultation services are not intended to replace the normal lines of communication among health care providers, residents, and families. But an ethics consult may be helpful when

- a resident, family member or health care provider wants help in "talking

  through" ethical issues involved in resident care;

- there is a serious ethical disagreement between health care providers, among family members, between health care providers and the resident, or between health care providers and family members;

- ethically, the case is unusual, unprecedented, or very complex;

- a resident, family member, or health care provider would like to have the

  benefit of other perspectives in working through an ethical problem.

Ethics consults are confidential. Any recommendations made are purely advisory in nature. Residents, family members, and health care providers remain responsible for making their own decisions. (5)

The importance that ethics committees have attained is indicated by mention of them as a mechanism for protecting resident rights in the standards for long-term care developed by the Joint Commission on Accreditation of Healthcare Organizations (JCAHO):

> The organization informs residents of their rights. The resident and his or her family have a way to question any suspected violation of their rights, for example, through an ethics committee or an individual(s) designed to handle ethical issues. [Intent of RI.1] (2)

Ethics committees began by focusing on issues in *clinical* practice. They discussed, for example, when it is permissible to withhold or withdraw tube feedings from residents. Some committees are expanding the scope of their activity to include *organizational* ethics. They are now considering "issues that previously were thought of as financial, administrative, organizational, or human resource questions." (6) In the future, ethics consults may be provided for the management of a health care facility just as ethics consults are now available to residents, family members, and staff for particular medical treatment decisions. (7)

Ethical Reasoning

This book uses many case studies describing concrete moral dilemmas in health care. Various exercises provide the opportunity to become involved in resolving these ethical dilemmas.

Some ethicists maintain that we can be sure only about general principles. When it comes to specific, concrete situations, we may never be one hundred percent certain about the right thing to do. This does not mean, however, that "anything goes" ethically in these situations. While ethical judgments may not reach certitude, this does not mean that they are arbitrary.

A good analogy for the type of ethical reasoning required is a jury trial. A jury is asked to determine if the defendant is guilty "beyond a reasonable doubt." Jury members are not asked to be one hundred percent certain that the defendant is guilty. Rather, they are asked to weigh the evidence for and against guilt and to determine if there are strong reasons for thinking the defendant is guilty. On this basis, the verdict is rendered and action is taken by the court.

Similarly, when someone tries to work through concrete ethical dilemmas in health care, she may find plausible reasons both for and against taking a particular course of action. But after weighing the ethical pros and cons, she needs to judge which course of action has the strongest reasons to support it and act on that basis. This is a very important point to keep in mind in "doing ethics" throughout this book.

NOTES

1. Diane E. Hoffmann, Philip Boyle & Steven A. Levenson, *Handbook for Nursing Home Ethics Committees* (Washington, DC: American Association of Homes and Services for the Aging, 1995).
2. Joint Commission on Accreditation of Healthcare Organizations, 2002-2003 *Standards for Long Term Care*, Resident Rights and Organization Ethics

(Oakbrook Terrace, IL: Joint Commission Resources, 2002).

3. Arthur L. Caplan, "The Morality of the Mundane: Ethical Issues Arising in the Daily Lives of Nursing Home Residents" in Rosalie A. Kane and Arthur L. Caplan (eds.), *Everyday Ethics Resolving Dilemmas in Nursing Home Life* (New York: Springer, 1990).

4. Judith Wilson Ross, *Handbook on Hospital Ethics Committees* (Chicago: American Hospital Publishing, 1986).

5. The information on ethics consultation is adapted from brochures prepared by the Clinical Ethics Committee of Mercy Medical Center, Dubuque, Iowa and the Medical Ethics Committee of the University of Nebraska Medical Center.

6. Judith Wilson Ross et al., *Health Care Ethics Committees The Next Generation* (Chicago: American Hospital Publishing, 1993).

7. American Society for Bioethics and Humanities, *Core Competencies for Health Care Ethics Consultation* (Glenview, IL: American Society for Bioethics and Humanities, 1998).

FOR FURTHER STUDY

- Diane E. Hoffmann, Philip Boyle, and Steven A. Levenson, *Handbook for Nursing Home Ethics Committees* (Washington, DC: American Association of Homes and Services for the Aging, 1995). This handbook provides extensive information on the practical aspects of setting up and sustaining an ethics committee.

- Dennis Brodeur, "Health Care Institutional Ethics: Broader Than Clinical Ethics" in John F. Monagle and David C. Thomasma (eds.), *Health Care Ethics: Critical Issues for the 21st Century* (Gaithersburg, MD: Aspen Publishers, 1998).

- Rosalie A. Kane and Arthur L. Caplan (eds.), *Everyday Ethics Resolving Dilemmas in Nursing Home Life* (New York: Springer, 1990).

- Mark P. Aulisio, Robert M. Arnold, and Stuart J. Younger, "Can There Be Educational and Training Standards for Those Conducting Health Care Ethics Consultation?" in John F. Monagle and David C. Thomasma (eds.), *Health Care Ethics: Critical Issues for the 21st Century* (Gaithersburg, MD: Aspen Publishers, 1998).

- American Society for Bioethics and Humanities, *Core Competencies for Health Care Ethics Consultation* (Glenview, IL: American Society for Bioethics and Humanities, 1998). This report discusses the nature and goals of ethics consultation and spells out very concretely specific skills and types of knowledge needed by an ethics consultation team. It also includes a chapter on organizational ethics.

Part One

Ethical Issues about Residency in a Long-Term Care Facility

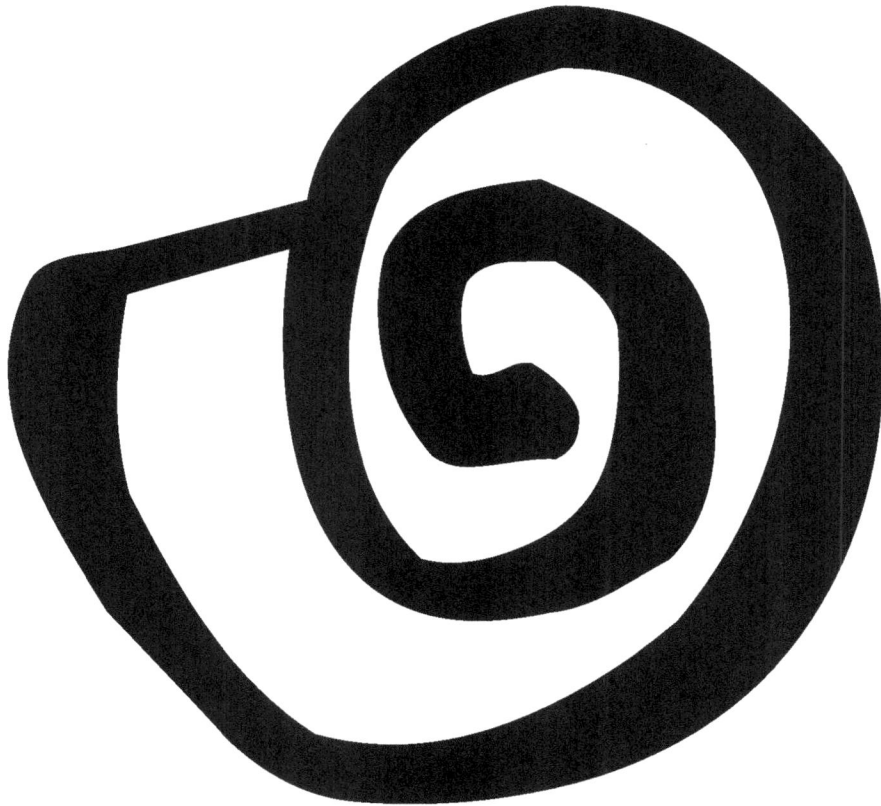

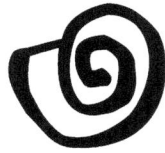

Chapter 2

Admissions Decisions

Admission to a long-term care facility is often an emotionally difficult time for the person who is becoming a resident. It may well mean giving up a home and familiar possessions. It means adjusting to an institutional environment and to living with complete strangers. Most of all, it involves a recognition that this will very probably be the last place of residence before death.

Admission to a long-term care facility can also be a difficult time for health care providers. The administrator of a long-term care facility may have to make choices among various individuals seeking admission. On the other hand, hospital discharge planners can be frustrated by difficulties in finding placement for patients ready to leave the hospital.

Ethical issues arise in the admissions process. Is it right to force an elderly parent to enter a long-term care facility against his will when others think this is for his own good? What kind of information about a potential resident can a facility expect to receive in the admissions process? When is it legitimate (and not discriminatory) to deny admission to a potential resident? If a facility is religiously sponsored, what role should religion play in the admission of residents?

This chapter covers:
- *the issue of who appropriately makes the decision to admit an individual to a long-term care facility;*
- *the role of the ethical principles of autonomy, nonmaleficence, truth-telling, and distributive justice in the admissions process;*
- *criteria that may be used in making admissions decisions.*

CASE STUDY
Virginia Nelson, 82, is a widow living alone at home. She has three children, two sons and one daughter, who are married and have families of their own. All of them still live in the same community, and they are devoted in visiting their mother and looking after her. They take turns in stopping by to check on their mother daily.

Virginia has occasional lapses of memory. Several times she has left an electric stove burner turned on for several hours, but nothing disastrous has happened—at least so far. In conversations, she tends to "live in the past." She does need some help with housekeeping, grocery shopping, and with bathing. But overall, she seems to be managing at home and to be quite content.

However, one morning her daughter Elaine stops by the house and finds her mother lying at the foot of the stairs. Apparently, her mother has fallen down the stairs.

Virginia seems confused, so that Elaine cannot find out exactly what happened or how long her mother has been lying there. Elaine drives her mother to the hospital emergency room, where she is diagnosed as having a concussion and a broken arm. Because of the concussion, she is admitted to the hospital until she regains mental lucidity.

That evening her three children have a family conference. They all feel that it is no longer safe for their mother to live alone. They decide to make arrangements for her to be placed in a long-term care facility when she is released from the hospital. They believe that their mother now needs someone with her all the time, and since the three of them and their spouses have full-time day jobs, they cannot provide the care their mother needs in their own homes.

The next day Elaine speaks with the administrator of Brookside Home, and fortunately, the facility has an immediate vacancy for her mother. Brookside Home has a reputation for being a quality long-term care facility, and Elaine has no qualms about promptly signing the admissions papers for her mother.

When Virginia is ready to be released from the hospital, her three children all go to see her to break the news about her transfer to the Brookside Home. When she finds out, Virginia starts crying. She protests that she doesn't need to go to a nursing home, and begs the nurses to call a taxi to take her home. Although Virginia's children feel badly about their mother's reaction, they believe their mother is not in a frame of mind to make a good decision about what is in her own best interests.

Autonomy in Admissions Decisions

A central principle in contemporary health care ethics is *autonomy*, or self-determination. Autonomy refers to the right of an individual to make the final decision in matters pertaining to his or her own life, including the realm of his or her health care. The admission of Virginia Nelson to a long-term care facility was handled in such a way as to violate her autonomy.

There are legitimate reasons for wondering if Virginia should continue to live at home alone. Her forgetfulness in leaving stove burners turned on is risky for her own safety since a fire could result. She has already been injured seriously enough by a fall down stairs to require hospitalization. Until Virginia's daughter found her, she was simply lying there, injured and mentally confused. Virginia's three children, who are devoted to looking after her, are undoubtedly thinking of her welfare in making arrangements for her admission to a long-term care facility. Surely, children do have an ethical obligation to try to prevent harm from coming to their elderly parents.

The problem lies in the fact that the children made the placement decision without consulting or involving their mother in any way. Indeed, Virginia was sent to the nursing home against her wishes. All of this violated Virginia's autonomy. It is true that Virginia has occasional lapses of memory and does much reminiscing about the past. However, this does not seem sufficient to disqualify her from having decision-making capacity. At the time that her children have a family conference to discuss her living arrangements, Virginia is still recovering from a concussion. The nursing home placement is not so urgent that the children could not wait until their mother has regained mental lucidity and this option could be discussed with her.

In reality, placement in a nursing home is often a group decision, involving not just the elderly person but also his or her family. (1) After all, these decisions affect the caregiving obligations and lives of the elderly person's family, not just the elderly person himself or herself. However, respect for the elderly person's autonomy requires that the decision be a mutual one between the elderly person and his or her family, not a unilateral decision by the family.

In speaking of the hospital discharge planning process for elderly patients, one author has commented:

> ...discharge planning decisions may affect the rights, duties, and obligations of family members. The decisions may require financial obligations. Families cannot unknowingly be enlisted in a discharge plan which requires their support and cannot be drafted into an unwilling army of caregivers. Nor, however, can they be permitted to coerce a patient into agreeing to a plan which is comfortable for them but unacceptable to the patient. The patient's desire and self-defined goal must be accommodated to family ability and willingness to help. Thus discharge planning often involves the reconciliation of the patient's and family's preferences. (2)

In the above case, a reconciliation must be achieved between Virginia's desire to remain in her own home and her children's ability to provide only limited care for her in that setting. Before Virginia is placed in a long-term care facility, other options might be considered for enhanced care for her, such as a live-in companion.

In the case of the admission of Virginia to Brookside Home, the administrator acted inappropriately in having her daughter, Elaine, sign the admissions agreement. Unfortunately, this has not been an uncommon practice:

> While there is currently more emphasis on active participation by older persons in the decision-making process, admissions staff sometimes prejudge the applicant's capacity for decision-making or accept the judgment of someone else that the applicant is "incompetent" to sign the admission contract. In the past, even competent persons have sometimes not been asked to sign their own contract... Facilities may insist on dealing with a family member or other "responsible party" who is the principal or only signer of the contract. Failure to involve a competent resident in the admissions process and subsequent treatment plan is a violation of federal laws and regulations. (1)

From an ethical point of view, such a practice is also a violation of a competent resident's autonomy.

In the above case, Virginia Nelson was discharged from a hospital to a nursing home. The following rules of thumb have been suggested to guide the discharge planning process for an elderly person from a hospital to other settings, including long-term care:

- Elderly persons who are capable of making decisions should be presented with the available options and should be given the opportunity to either consent to or refuse the various alternatives.

- Decisionally capable elderly persons have the right to assume personal risks even if those risks may place them in a situation of potential harm. The choice of risk does not negate the person being decisionally capable.

- Caregivers have the responsibility to discuss with decisionally capable elderly persons which alternative is considered in the person's best medical interest and which ones are realistically feasible, given family and community supports.

- Elderly persons of diminished, uncertain or fluctuating decisional capacity may still be able to participate in the decision making process and may be able to select an option according to their own personal desires and values. Caregivers should discuss options with such persons at times when the person's decision making capability is most intact.

- Given the variety of factors involved in developing a discharge plan, family members or other close individuals should be encouraged (after the consent of the person in question has been obtained) to participate in the discharge-planning process and to assist that person in selecting a discharge option. It should be made clear to all participants, however, that the choice is first and foremost that of the elderly person himself or herself.

- Efforts should be made to educate family members regarding the availability of community supports and reimbursement mechanisms that could ease the obligations or burdens which they may face as a result of the discharge plan. (2)

These rules of thumb could also be used in making decisions about long-term care placement directly from the home setting. Ethically, it should be noted that the first, second, fourth, and fifth guidelines reflect the principle of autonomy.

CASE STUDY

Since the death of his wife a year ago, Wayne Morgan, 75, has been living with his oldest son, Tom, Tom's wife, Gini, and their two teenage children. After the death of his mother, Tom brought up the idea of his dad getting a small apartment. However, Wayne has never done cooking or housework, and doesn't feel he can manage on his own. As he says, "you can't teach an old dog new tricks."

Through his business partner Tom knows the administrator of the Woodstock Care Center, Don Moser. Tom decides to speak with Don about placing his father at Woodstock. Tom tells Don that his father is incontinent, has real difficulty walking, and is becoming increasingly forgetful. For these reasons, he is reluctant to leave his father alone at home, which must sometimes be done because of his own work schedule and that of his wife and because of the activities of their children. Tom indicates that his father has the money to pay his own way at the nursing home.

Woodstock Care Center requires a pre-admission interview with any potential resident who is still mentally competent, and Don Moser agrees to interview Wayne Morgan. At the interview Wayne indicates that his son has spoken with him about moving to Woodstock Care Center, and that he is willing to do this. Wayne says that he feels he has become a burden on Tom, Gini, and his grandchildren. "They have their own lives to live," he says, and "I don't want to interfere."

In conversation Don Moser finds Wayne to be very lucid mentally. Don also learns that Wayne is still able to do some work in the garden at home and that he occasionally plays golf. Wayne states that his major complaint is arthritis, for which he may eventually need knee replacement surgery.

After this interview, Don Moser has doubts that Wayne really needs nursing home placement at the present time. He sees discrepancies between Tom's description of his father's condition and the man he saw at the interview. Don wonders what family dynamics may underlie Tom's push for nursing home placement for his dad.

Questionable Admissions

In the previous case about Virginia Nelson, we saw that her autonomy was violated in the way her placement in a long-term care facility was handled. Unlike Virginia, Wayne Morgan is willing to enter a long-term care facility. And unlike the case of Virginia whose children unilaterally made the decision to place her in a nursing home, Wayne's son talked with him about moving to Woodstock Care Center. Prima facie, Wayne's autonomy seemed to be respected in the admissions process. However, in his case more subtle pressures may be at work to erode his autonomous decision making.

After the pre-admission interview, the administrator of Woodstock Care Center wonders what family dynamics may underlie the push for nursing home placement for Wayne Morgan on the part of his son. Indeed, during the pre-admission interview Wayne says that he feels he has become a burden on his son and his family, and expresses a desire not to interfere in their lives. Is the son's house too small to accommodate Wayne comfortably? Does Wayne feel that he is getting in the way? Do his teenage grandchildren feel that his presence is dampening their socialization with friends in their own home? Are there conflicts between Wayne and his daughter-in-law? Is Wayne left out of the family's activities? If Wayne feels unwelcome in his son's home, this can pressure him to choose nursing home placement.

While it is true that Wayne's son discussed placement at the Woodstock Care Center with him, it can also happen that such family discussions are skewed:

> Families sometimes manipulate their elder members into believing that a nursing home or other living arrangement is needed. ...They will offer false reassurances and optimistic statements about living in a facility. Family members may try to have the older person assessed during a "visit" and pressure the elder member to see nursing home life in positive terms. (1)

While Wayne says that he is willing to move to Woodstock Care Center, it is questionable that his condition warrants placement in a long-term care facility. After all, he is still able to do some work in the garden at home and even occasionally plays golf. Has his son effectually talked Wayne into this move?

This case also raises the ethical issue of truth-telling. The administrator of Woodstock Care Center notes discrepancies between the description of Wayne's condition given by his son and what he himself perceives during the pre-admission interview with Wayne. In this instance, the son portrays his father's condition as being worse than it in fact is. Unfortunately, children giving an inaccurate picture of a parent's condition to ensure nursing home placement happens all too frequently:

> Family members may also shade the truth or give an incomplete picture of the older person's capacities. "Sure, Mother can dress herself." They may over- or underplay the true status of their family member depending on what they believe will help get their member admitted. Other professionals may reinforce this falsification. Doctors, lawyers, clergy, and friends may tell the admissions staff that the older person meets admission requirements when, in fact, there may be discrepancies in behaviors and abilities. (1)

It is important that long-term care facilities be given accurate information about a potential resident's condition for several reasons. First of all, a facility should be able to provide the level and kind of care a particular person needs; if not, the individual may suffer harm. Indeed, suitability for the particular facility is one principle which should guide admissions decisions:

> Preference should be given to those patients who can best be cared for with the services and staff currently available at the facility. Those needing a higher or lower level of care should be directed elsewhere... (3)

Second, decisions about who is admitted to a facility are decisions about the allocation of health care resources. Admitting one individual may well mean denying access to another. It is questionable that Wayne Morgan needs nursing home care at this point in his life. Admitting him to the Woodstock Care Center may mean denying admission to someone who really does need that level of care. Ethically, we want to say that this is unfair. More formally stated, admitting Wayne Morgan would represent a violation of the principle of distributive justice; that is, the principle of fairness in the distribution of benefits and resources.

CASE STUDY

Ray Miller, 76, is taken to the Emergency Room of Lakeview Community Hospital after falling down the basement stairs at home. He suffers from mild dementia. Ray is diagnosed as having a broken hip, which is surgically repaired. Ray is also found to have an infection, and antibiotic treatment is promptly begun. The infection proves to be antibiotic resistant, but fortunately, it seems to run its course.

A decision is made to transfer Ray to a nursing home. Ray's wife, Alice, suffers from a serious heart condition and the caregiving strains associated with Ray's recovery from hip surgery might be too much for her. Ray's three children all live out of state, so they cannot offer Alice any day-to-day help with caregiving. And then there is the problem of Ray's dementia.

Megan McCormick is the social worker assigned to assist with Ray's discharge planning. There are three long-term care facilities in the community that she can contact.

Megan first calls the Mississippi Valley Care Center. She describes Ray's condition to the administrator, and is honest about the fact that Ray has recently experienced an infection that is resistant to antibiotics. The administrator tells Megan that the facility cannot provide the level of care that Ray really needs. Ray ought to be placed in a private room for the sake of infection control, the administrator explains, but the facility currently has only double rooms available.

Megan then contacts the Oak Ridge Home, again describing Ray's condition to the facility's administrator. The administrator responds that Ray couldn't possibly be admitted at the present time because of the facility's waiting list.

Finally, Megan calls the Hillcrest Care Center. Initially, the administrator seems quite receptive to admitting Ray. But when she finds out that Ray has recently experienced an infection resistant to antibiotics, Megan notices that her attitude changes. The administrator tells Megan that she will have to "do some checking" before she can finally admit Ray. The next day Megan receives a message from Hillcrest indicating that the facility will be unable to admit Ray. No reason is given.

A week goes by and the administration of Lakeview Community Hospital begins to put pressure on Megan to find some placement for Ray. In frustration, Megan contacts the Glen Haven Care Center, located in a small community forty miles away. This time she tells them only about Ray's broken hip. Glen Haven will accept Ray, and Megan begins the procedures for Ray's transfer to that facility. At the same time, she is not entirely comfortable with this transfer. Glen Haven is not of the same quality as the three nursing homes within the local community. Besides, Ray's wife will not be able to visit him very often because of the location of Glen Haven.

Denying Admission

This case is written from the perspective of a hospital discharge planner, and illustrates the frustration such individuals can experience in working with nursing homes. Certain types of patients can be notoriously difficult to place in long-term care facilities; for example, persons who have a history of aggressive or disruptive behavior, persons with an alcohol problem, and persons who require heavy and/or expensive care. (1) In the case at hand, Ray is hard to place because he has recently suffered an infection resistant to antibiotics—a new problem in health care.

This case also illustrates the pressures which today are being put on hospital discharge planners to discharge patients to nursing homes as quickly as possible. (1) Indeed, because of this pressure the social worker assigned to assist with Ray Miller's discharge planning suppresses information about his condition in order to achieve placement in a nursing home. This again raises the ethical issue of truthtelling, and concomitantly, of the right of long-term care facilities to have accurate and complete information about potential residents. But above all, this case raises the issue of fairness in admission to long-term care facilities. What reasons for denying admission to a particular person are legitimate ones? And what reasons are illegitimate and discriminatory?

In the case of Hillcrest Care Center, it seems clear that Ray is denied admission just because he has recently experienced an infection resistant to antibiotics. It should be noted that an Antibiotic Resistance Task Force in the State of Iowa has concluded "admission to licensed facilities should not be denied because the patient is colonized or infected with an antibiotic resistant organism." (4) Although no particular reason is given why Ray is denied admission at Hillcrest, one can speculate about possible causes.

Just as occurred in the case of AIDS, there may be a fear that other residents will become infected with antibiotic resistant organisms. This would be especially frightening if a facility has not yet had a resident with an antibiotic resistant infection. An administrator might feel that exposing current residents to this risk would be unfair to them. Ethically, health care workers have a duty of nonmaleficence, that is, a duty to prevent harm from coming to patients and residents.

However, denying admission to Ray on this basis would be due to ignorance on the part of the administrator and staff of Hillcrest Care Center. Just as the spread of the AIDS virus can be controlled, so the spread of antibiotic resistant organisms can be controlled through use of the appropriate infection control procedures. (4) The principle of nonmaleficence is not appropriately applied here to deny admission to Ray.

The administrator of the Mississippi Valley Care Center does not want to accept Ray because "the facility cannot provide the level of care that Ray really needs." If true, this certainly seems like a legitimate reason to deny admission to a facility. (1, 3) Accepting an individual under these circumstances would pose a threat of harm to the person himself or herself, violating the health care worker's ethical duty of nonmaleficence.

However, one can question the factual accuracy of the administrator's judgment that the facility cannot provide the level of care that Ray needs. The administrator states "Ray ought to be placed in a private room for the sake of infection control" but that "the facility currently has only double rooms available." Specifically on the issue of private rooms and roommates, the Iowa Antibiotic Resistance Task Force reached these conclusions:

> Private rooms are always ideal, but in most long term care facilities the number of private rooms is limited. Transmission of these bacteria between roommates is uncommon where colonization or infection with controlled drainage, etc., is present. Therefore, routinely placing patients into a private room is not warranted. (4)

Further, a long-term care facility can "cohort residents who are colonized or infected with the same organism." (4) To maintain appropriate infection control, a facility can also avoid placing residents with antibiotic resistant organisms "with other residents who have indwelling tubes, Stage III or IV decubitus ulcers, deep open wounds, multiple functional disabilities, or are receiving long-term antimicrobial agents." (4) Thus, the Mississippi Valley Care Center ought to be willing to accept Ray as a resident.

Moreover, we are told that Ray's infection seems to have run its course. Cultures can and should be taken to determine Ray's current status and whether anything beyond standard infection control precautions are still needed for him. (4)

Finally, the Oak Ridge Home declines to accept Ray because the facility already has people on a waiting list. One principle that long-term care facilities can adopt for making admissions decisions is "first come, first served":

> This is the principle of pure equality, which refuses to consider such factors as individual needs, availability of financial resources or consequences for the institution. Instead, a waiting list is established, and admission is strictly according to the list. (3)

The "first come, first served" principle embodies the ethical value of egalitarianism (3), and is a familiar principle in American society. If this principle indeed represents the policy of the Oak Ridge Home, then Ray Miller was not treated unfairly in being denied admission.

A question might be raised, however, whether a "first come, first served" policy is the best way to make admissions decisions. Should someone's ranking on a waiting list be weighed against other factors? (3) Other principles that may be used in making admissions decisions will be explored in the next section.

CASE STUDY

The Pleasantville Presbyterian Home is located in a small, rural Midwestern community. It is the only long-term care facility located within a forty-mile radius. The home has a committee to help the facility's administrator deal with particularly difficult admissions decisions. The admissions committee is comprised of the administrator and the facility's director of nursing, social worker, and chaplain.

At present, there is one private room available due to the recent death of a resident. The administrator brings to the committee the persons whom she considers the three top candidates for admission.

The first is Jeanne Kraus, aged 80. Mrs. Kraus is ambulatory, but needs substantial assistance in taking care of herself and is no longer capable of living alone at home. Mrs. Kraus has been a devout Presbyterian all her life, and her daughter has contacted the Pleasantville Presbyterian Home precisely because it has a resident chaplain and holds various religious services several times a week. The daughter believes that her mother would fit in much better at this facility than a nondenominational home because of its active religious life. Mrs. Kraus has the financial resources to pay her own way.

The second candidate is the mother of John Miller. Ten years ago John's parents moved to Arizona for retirement. Mrs. Miller, aged 76, is now a widow and needs nursing home care because of a chronic illness. John wants to relocate his mother to the geographical area in which he lives so that she can be with family and have their support. John has done much volunteer work for the Pleasantville Presbyterian Home. In fact, he has headed several very successful fund drives for the facility.

The third candidate is Stephen Young, 68, who is scheduled to be discharged from the hospital. Although still ambulatory at the present time, Mr. Young has pancreatic cancer and is expected to die within six months. His wife died several years ago, and his two children were killed in their teens in a boating accident. His brothers and their families all live out of state. Since Mr. Young has no one to take care of him at home, he is seeking nursing home placement. Mr. Young could benefit greatly from the facility's hospice program. However, Mr. Young would be on Medicaid, and the payments from this governmental program would fall substantially short of the actual cost of his care.

The Pleasantville Presbyterian Home could provide the level of care needed by any of these persons. The question is, which one should be admitted?

Selecting Among Applicants for Admission

Thus far we have encountered several principles which may be used in making admissions decisions: first come, first served on a waiting list; whether the facility can provide the level of care which the prospective resident needs; the risks which would be posed to current residents by the prospective admission. Analyzing the dilemma faced by the Pleasantville Presbyterian Home will uncover additional considerations that may figure into admissions decisions.

Clearly, one consideration is financial. Mrs. Kraus would be "private pay," because she has the personal financial resources to cover the cost of her care in a long-term care facility. Mr. Young, on the other hand, would be on Medicaid, a governmental program with reimbursements often below the actual cost of care. In fact, it is stated that Pleasantville Presbyterian Home will lose money by admitting Mr. Young.

Surely, administrators of long-term care facilities and admissions committees have an ethical responsibility to maintain the economic viability of the facility. If they do not do this, then the facility may have to close, with serious hardships being imposed on current residents. At the same time many long-term care facilities, especially those that are not-for-profit and religiously sponsored, see it as part of their mission to provide care for those in need. Indeed, such facilities may engage in fund raising specifically to subsidize the care of residents whose own financial resources are exhausted.

These two ethical commitments—maintaining a facility's financial viability and providing care for individuals in need independent of their ability to pay—are sometimes reconciled by a facility deciding upon a payer mix, in which a certain percentage of its beds (and only this percentage) are allocated to Medicaid residents. Under this kind of policy, the eligibility of Mr. Young for admission would depend upon the number of current residents on Medicaid at Pleasantville Presbyterian Home.

This case also raises the question of the role of institutional culture in admissions decisions. Mrs. Kraus' daughter is exploring admission to the Pleasantville Presbyterian Home for her mother precisely because her mother is a devout Presbyterian and this home provides that type of religious environment. In the case of John Miller's mother and Stephen Young, we have no indication whether the religious affiliation of the home plays a role in the decision to seek admission or whether admission is being sought simply because this is the only long-term care facility in a forty-mile radius. Should Mrs. Kraus receive preference in admission to this facility because her own religious affiliation matches that of the home?

The answer to this question is related to the stated mission of the institution. Compare the following mission statements of two religiously sponsored facilities:

> Residents are admitted without regard to race, creed, religion, color, sex, or national origin.

> The primary purpose of Tel Yehuda Home shall be to establish environments for aged Jewish persons which will provide for their health and well-being and in which they will be encouraged and assisted in fulfilling their own social and spiritual needs and practicing their own culture and religious traditions. (1)

The second mission statement would allow preference being given to prospective residents of a particular religious affiliation whereas the first one would not. Giving such preference would be analogous to what occurs at veterans' hospitals. It is the explicit mission of a veterans' hospital to serve the health care needs of veterans of the armed forces, and such a mission is regarded by our society as a legitimate one. Hence, it is not unfair for someone who is not a veteran to be excluded from services at such a hospital.

The role that religious affiliation may legitimately play in admissions decisions to long-term care facilities is summarized well in this way:

> Depending on the mission of the facility, as stated in official documents, admission decisions may include or exclude religious affiliation. Non-public institutions are free to decide what their missions are. If they state that they will accept all without regard to race, creed, color, etc., then they may not discriminate on any of those bases. If they use a narrower standard such as religious affiliation, then this information must be publicly stated and communicated to any applicants. (1)

The decision about admitting John Miller's mother also involves the issue of constituencies served by a particular facility. Since Mrs. Miller is living in Arizona, she is outside the geographical service area of the Pleasantville Presbyterian Home. Further, it was by their own choice that Mr. and Mrs. Miller moved to Arizona. Should preference be given to applicants from the facility's service area? (3)

In support of an affirmative response, it might be pointed out that the local community may well provide various kinds of support for the home. For example, community members may volunteer in various ways at the home, or fund raising for the home may take place within the community. If one is dealing with a public (versus a private) facility, members of the community support the facility through taxes. It can be argued that such activities create an obligation for the facility to serve the members of the constituency who make possible its continued existence.

However, it is stated that John Miller himself "has done much volunteer work" for the home and that "he has headed several very successful fund drives for the facility." Has this not created an obligation on the part of the facility to John Miller? (3) Certainly, the facility owes John a debt of gratitude. Does not this debt of gratitude create a point in favor of admitting his mother?

Further, maintaining family integrity and supporting family caregiving are values that a long-term care facility may wish to support:

> The integrity of the family would support preferential admission for the spouse of a current resident or for those with community-residing family caregivers who can maintain ties after admission, for example, because of proximity to the facility. (3)

It should be noted that John Miller wants his mother placed in the Pleasantville Presbyterian Home so that "she can be with family and have their support."

Finally, there is Stephen Young to consider. Yet another principle that may be used in the admissions process is to "select the neediest first." (3) This principle favors "admitting those who are sickest, those with the worst prognosis, those least able to care for themselves at home or those with the shortest life expectancy." (3) Among the three candidates for admission, it is Stephen Young who is terminally ill with pancreatic cancer and has a life expectancy of only six months. Hospice services would be available to him at the nursing home, but he could not stay at home to receive hospice care since he has no home caregivers available. His wife and children are deceased, and his brothers all live out of state. Admitting Mr. Young to the Pleasantville Presbyterian Home would provide a much needed support system for him during his dying process.

In sum, we have identified in the course of this chapter the following criteria that may enter into admissions decisions:

- Do the needs of the prospective resident match the kind and level of care that the facility is able to provide?
- Will the admission of the prospective resident pose any risks to current residents?
- What is the position of the prospective resident on a waiting list?
- What impact will the admission of the prospective resident have on the financial viability of the facility?
- Does the prospective resident fit the articulated mission of the facility?
- Is the prospective resident from the constituency which, broadly understood, provides support for the facility?

- Will admission of the prospective resident promote family integrity and caregiving?

- How needy is the prospective resident in comparison with other potential residents?

These are presented as *possible* criteria to use, and are listed without any intended rank order. However, they should provide a basis for reflection in formulating admissions policy within a particular facility.

Joint Commission Standards

The standards for long-term care developed by the Joint Commission on Accreditation of Healthcare Organizations (JCAHO) include the area of admissions. Related to the cases we have considered, there are several noteworthy points. A facility's preadmission process should include defined categories of individuals who are and are not accepted by the facility (e.g., individuals undergoing chemotherapy), and established criteria to determine admission eligibility [Intent of CC.2.1]. (6) A facility should accept individuals only when their assessed needs can be met [Intent of CC.2]. If an individual is denied admission following the preadmission screening, the reasons for denying admission should be stated [Intent of CC.2.1]. (6) Further, in such a case staff should make reasonable efforts to refer the individual to another appropriate organization [Intent of CC.2.1]. (6)

FOR GROUP DISCUSSION

1. Have you ever been in the position of having a mentally competent family member admitted to a long-term care facility? Reflect on how the admissions process was handled from an ethical point of view. In particular, was the autonomy of the family member respected during the admissions process?

2. One complaint about the admissions process has been the use of admissions agreements that are hard for prospective residents to read because of the use of small print, complicated sentence structure, and technical, legal language. (1,5) Such documents erode a prospective resident's autonomy in making a choice about a long-term care facility. If you are connected with a long-term care facility, review the admissions agreement used by the facility from this perspective. (If you are not connected with a long-term care facility, you might still obtain such a contract from a local facility and review it.)

3. If you are connected with a long-term care facility, find out if the facility has an explicit set of admissions standards. How do these standards compare with possible criteria identified in this chapter?

4. Consider the list of possible criteria for admissions decisions. Which criteria would you personally use, and why? Would you eliminate any of the listed criteria? Are there any other criteria you would add to the list? If necessary, how would you prioritize the criteria you have selected?

5. If you are connected with a long-term care facility, read the facility's mission statement and determine what implications it has for admissions decisions.

6. Consider the case involving the Pleasantville Presbyterian Home. Suppose you are a member of the admissions committee. Whom would you choose to admit? What factors are significant in reaching your decision? (Various individuals might role-play the discussion of the admissions committee.)

NOTES

1. Robert L. Schneider, *The Admissions Process: Nursing Homes and Ethical Issues* (Washington, DC: American Association of Homes and Services for the Aging, 1994).
2. Nancy Neveloff Dubler, "Improving the Discharge Planning Process: Distinguishing Between Coercion and Choice," *The Gerontologist* 28 Suppl. (1998): 76-81.
3. Harry R. Moody, "Some Principles Governing Equitable Nursing Home Access" in Rosalie A. Kane and Arthur L. Caplan (eds.), *Everyday Ethics Resolving Dilemmas in Nursing Home Life* (New York: Springer, 1990).
4. *Report of the Iowa Antibiotic Resistance Task Force*, "Guidelines for Long Term Care Facility" (Des Moines, IA: Iowa Antibiotic Resistance Task Force, 1999).
5. Donna Myers Ambrogi and Frances Leonard, "The Impact of Nursing Home Admission Agreements on Resident Autonomy," *The Gerontologist* 28 Suppl. (1988): 82-89.
6. Joint Commission on Accreditation of Healthcare Organizations, 2002-2003 *Standards for Long Term Care* (Oakbrook Terrace, IL: Joint Commission Resources, 2002).

FOR FURTHER STUDY

*   Donna Myers Ambrogi, "Nursing Home Admissions: Problematic Process and Agreements," *Generations* 14 Suppl. (1990): 72-74.

*   Charles P. Sabatino, "Nursing Home Admission Contracts: Undermining Rights the Old-Fashioned Way," *Clearinghouse Review* 24 (Oct. 1990): 553-56.

*   H.R. Moody, "Ethical Dilemmas in Nursing Home Placement," *Generations* 11/4 (Summer 1987): 16-23.

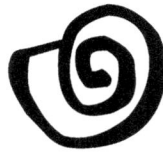

Chapter 3

Decisions about Transferring and Relocating Residents

Once an individual has been admitted to a long-term care facility, this does not necessarily mean that there will be no further decisions to be made concerning the place of residency. Especially with the increasing number of multi-level complexes for older adults, ranging from independent living apartments to assisted living to various levels of nursing home care, decisions will have to be made about transferring a resident from one level to another. A resident may also be faced with the possibility of relocating to another facility, perhaps because a child who is the primary caregiver is moving to another community. Transfer and relocation can also take place because of financial considerations.

This chapter covers:
* *factors which make it difficult for residents to transfer to a higher level of care within a facility;*
* *ethical principles involved in such transfer decisions;*
* *the role of financial considerations in placing and relocating residents in long-term care facilities;*
* *the concept of a right to health care.*

CASE STUDY

Millie Taylor is a resident of the Oak Ridge Baptist Home, a multi-level facility. Millie has been residing in one of the assisted living apartments for three years. During this time, she has remained active, and has even served as the resident representative on the facility's ethics committee. Millie was a music teacher for many years, and she has in her apartment an extensive collection of records, tapes, and compact disks. Listening to music is one of her favorite pastimes.

Within the last six months, however, Millie's health has begun to decline. Her eyesight in particular has become very poor. She is stumbling over objects and furniture in her apartment, and sometimes she cannot see well enough to be sure that she has turned off appliances. The staff of Oak Ridge is concerned about her safety. They think it would be best if she moved to the nursing home section of the facility, where more help and supervision are available.

When the director of nursing (DON) approaches Millie about the move, Millie becomes quite upset. She protests that she doesn't want to make the move. The apartment is "her home," and besides, she wouldn't be able to take her music collection with her to the other section. "I don't know what I would do without my music," she says.

Transfer to Another Level of Care

In this case, Millie Taylor resists the recommendation of the director of nursing to transfer to another section of the facility providing a higher level of care. The staff is concerned about her safety in the apartment, and undoubtedly they are thinking of her welfare in suggesting the move.

However, there are several reasons why Millie may find the move to the nursing home section of the facility to be difficult.

First, there is the phenomenon of "place bonding":

> ...as persons develop a sense of place over time, they attach special meaning to certain activities and events that are strongly identified with particular spaces. This process is known as place bonding. While it is easy to understand that older persons bond with their homes and all their personal possessions, it is important to know that older persons will bond with an apartment, room, corridor or even a window with a certain view. Relocation or transfer from any place to which an older person is bonded will cause a sense of displacement with a resulting sense of loss. (1)

It should be noted that Millie describes the apartment she has in the facility as "her home."

Second, the nursing home section of the Oak Ridge Baptist Home will undoubtedly be an environment in which Millie's activities are more restricted than in the apartment setting. This loss of choice and control will also make the move difficult:

> Another particular characteristic of relocation of older persons is an inevitable loss of autonomy. Along with the personal bonding to a place, older persons have a sense of control and freedom to choose how to live out their daily lives. There is probably no other place where individuals can feel more in charge of their lives than in their homes, apartments or rooms. If a change or relocation from this environment is required, there is usually a change in the level of autonomy, frequently downward with fewer choices and less control. As one resident...said, "I may have to move to the [health care] center and then I *will have less to say about what I do, where I go and who I see...*" (1)

Third, transfer from one level of care to a higher one within a facility is psychologically difficult because it forces the resident to recognize declining health status and is a reminder of his or her eventual death:

> Acknowledging a change in one's health status is not an easy task for most persons, and it is frequently accompanied by a strong sense of denial and delay. Facing even a reversible condition requires fortitude because the condition reminds the person of his or her mortality. The sequence of events that inevitably flows from a change in health status is crystallized in the concrete act of moving from one place to another. Relocation thus

represents a dynamic dimension of living and dying that is not easily accepted. (1)

Family members will sometimes oppose the transfer of a resident to a higher level of care. One factor that may be operating is the difficulty family members also experience in recognizing and accepting the declining health status of a spouse or a parent.

Finally, in Millie's case there is another factor that will make the move difficult. Millie was a music teacher by profession, and she still has an extensive collection of records, tapes, and compact disks with her in the apartment. She will not be able to take this collection of music with her to the nursing home section of the facility. This will represent loss of part of her personal identity. As Millie states, "I don't know what I would do without my music."

From an ethical point of view, the case of Millie Taylor is a classic case of conflict between two ethical principles: autonomy and nonmaleficence. *Autonomy* refers to self-determination. In a health care context, it refers to the right of a patient or resident to make the final decision in matters pertaining to his or her own life and health care. *Nonmaleficence* is the duty of a health care worker to prevent harm from coming to patients and residents. According to the principle of autonomy, Millie should be allowed to assume the risks of remaining in her apartment if that is her choice. The duty of nonmaleficence, on the other hand, requires the facility's staff to do everything in their power to effect Millie's transfer to the nursing home unit in order to prevent injury to her.

In addition, the ethical principle of *distributive justice* is relevant to this case. Distributive justice concerns fairness in the distribution of benefits, burdens, and resources. An assisted living apartment no longer fits Millie's needs. If Millie remains in the apartment rather than going to the nursing home unit, she may well be taking this place in the facility away from someone for whom an assisted living apartment represents the exact level of care that is presently needed. Allowing Millie to remain in the apartment would seem to be an inappropriate use of the facility's resources.

How should this situation be handled? Some facilities have in place a policy reserving to the facility the right to make the final transfer decision. (1) However, out of respect for Millie's autonomy, the staff of Oak Ridge Baptist Home ought first to seek to obtain her agreement to the move. Since she is mentally competent, they should speak with her and present the reasons why they think it is advisable for her to move to the nursing home unit of the home.

Indeed, the ethically right thing to do is reinforced by legal considerations. From the perspective of due process, questions can be raised whether a facility has given adequate time for communication, meetings, and negotiation in transfer and relocation decisions. (1)

The staff of the home could try to ease the transition for Millie by seeing what cherished objects from her current apartment could be put in her new room (e.g., a favorite chair, an heirloom clock). Indeed, the standards for long-term care developed by the Joint Commission on Accreditation of Healthcare Organizations (JCAHO) recommend that "residents' living space contain items, such as pictures, clothing, photos, radios, furniture, afghans, and the like, that help them personalize the space" [Intent of RI.2.11]. (2) This would help minimize the sense of displacement. While Millie's music collection undoubtedly could not be placed in her new room, perhaps arrangements could be made for her to have access to it in a lounge area of the home.

The case as described above represents Millie's initial reaction to the idea of being transferred to the nursing home unit. If Millie is given reasons why the transfer is advisable, given time to think it over, and the aforementioned accommodations are offered to her, perhaps she will be willing to agree to the move.

CASE STUDY

Dorothy and Leo Hansen, both 84, have been residents of the Hawthorne Lake Care Center for three years. This facility has a reputation for providing exceptionally good care and accommodations for its residents.

Because of their declining health and their advanced age when they had to enter a nursing home, Dorothy and Leo really didn't expect to live all that much longer. They chose Hawthorne Lake Care Center, even though it is somewhat expensive, because they wanted to spend the time remaining to them as comfortably and enjoyably as they could. After working hard all their lives and raising five children, they felt they owed something to themselves.

Hawthorne Lake Care Center accepts as residents only those individuals who are private pay. In living longer than they expected, Dorothy and Leo have exhausted their own savings and must now depend on Medicaid to cover the cost of their care. They have been informed by the Hawthorne Lake Care Center that they will have to move to another facility. They have been notified that they must move within a month.

Relocation to Another Facility

It goes without saying that relocating to another facility will be traumatic for Dorothy and Leo Hansen. After three years of residency at the Hawthorne Lake Care Center, years which presumably have been enjoyable ones for them, they have undoubtedly bonded to the facility. They will have to leave the friends they have made at the facility. At the age of 84, the mere fact of moving to another location will be difficult. Further, they have only a month in which to find another placement. Given the waiting lists that often exist for admission to good facilities, will they be able to find a satisfactory placement in time? Where will they go, if they do not? Will they have increased difficulty in finding placement because they are Medicaid recipients? Will they be forced to move to a geographical area which distances them from their children?

From an ethical point of view, are Dorothy and Leo being treated unfairly in being required to move out of the Hawthorne Lake Care Center? There are some facilities that guarantee lifetime occupancy to prospective residents. However, such facilities frequently require a transfer of substantial assets in return. (3) We have no indication that Dorothy and Leo were admitted to this care center under these conditions. Certainly, it is a matter of fairness that prospective residents be advised at the time of admission if the facility has a "private pay only" policy. If this was in fact done by the Hawthorne Lake Care Center and Dorothy and Leo accepted residency under these conditions, then some would argue that they have no grounds for complaint in being asked to relocate at this time.

However, a more fundamental question may be asked: Is it legitimate for facilities to have a policy of restricting their services to private pay residents? What justifications might be offered by the Hawthorne Lake Care Center for having only residents who can pay their own way?

First of all, this care center is recognized as a facility that provides "exceptionally good care and accommodations for its residents." Maintaining this high quality of service entails significant costs. In the case of Medicaid, reimbursement rates are usually below what facilities need to charge in order to balance costs with income. (4) Hence, Hawthorne Lake Care Center might argue that private pay residents are needed to maintain the quality of the institution.

Further, this facility may be reluctant to accept Medicaid residents because some persons deliberately transfer their assets just to qualify for Medicaid and to avoid personal payment to the facility. (4) Ethically, this practice is problematic in "siphoning off resources" from the poor who are the intended recipients of the Medicaid program. (4) From a practical point of view, this practice creates financial strains for the facility because of the low Medicaid reimbursement rates.

In addition, facilities may find participation in the Medicaid system downright burdensome (3):

> ...it is their perception of being enmeshed in a bureaucratic straitjacket that explains why nursing homes desire to extricate themselves from Medicaid involvement. Because it is costly, time-consuming, and frustrating to comply with Medicaid regulations, they have a strong inducement to opt out. (3)

In sum, the choice of a facility to be exclusively private pay may be related to flaws in the Medicaid system; namely, unrealistically low reimbursement rates, bureaucratic red tape, and abuses in its use.

Although Dorothy and Leo Hansen freely chose to reside at the Hawthorne Lake Care Center, we may still have a nagging doubt that it was really fair for them to undergo the trauma of relocation at their age. If we intuitively feel that something is ethically amiss, then we should look to systemic reform of health care financing for the elderly. Thus, a case of relocating a couple to another facility has brought us into the realm of social justice and social ethics.

It has become popular to claim that people have a *right* to health care. (5, 6) However, this right is often interpreted as a claim on certain basic services, not necessarily all possible health care services or the very best health care services that are available. (5, 6) Hawthorne Lake Care Center is described as "providing exceptionally good care and accommodations for its residents." Some might argue that the right which Dorothy and Leo have to health care does not necessarily entitle them to residency at a facility of the caliber of Hawthorne Lake, but that their right may be satisfied by residency at a facility which provides "a decent level of care." (3)

This type of response challenges us to consider a very fundamental question about our ethical obligations to older persons. In view of the contributions the elderly have made to the society we now enjoy, what kind and quality of care do we owe them?

Joint Commission Standards

Medical reasons, the welfare of the resident, the welfare of other residents, or non-payment of fees are recognized by the Joint Commission on Accreditation of Healthcare Organizations (JCAHO) as legitimate reasons for transferring or discharging a resident [Intent of RI.4]. (2) This includes room-to-room transfers [Intent of RI.4]. (2) A facility should not only provide a resident with notice of the transfer or discharge, but an explanation of the need for it and relevant policies of the facility [Intent of RI.4]. (2) JCAHO standards urge a facility to consider the effect of a transfer on a resident, and caution that multiple transfers of residents ought to be avoided [Intent of RI.4]. (2)

FOR GROUP DISCUSSION

1. If you work at a long-term care facility, review any policies the facility has in place with respect to the transfer of residents within the facility. How do these policies compare with points made in this chapter? Do the policies embody a respect for the autonomy of residents? Do the policies place a priority on preventing harm from coming to residents or on resident autonomy? Upon reflection, do you think that the facility's policies should be modified in any way? (If you do not work at a long-term care facility, you might interview staff at such a facility about these issues.)

2. Consider the case of Millie Taylor. Suppose that staff has talked with her about the reasons favoring transfer to the nursing home unit of the facility and has tried to accommodate her possessions and interests in the new setting, but that Millie still persists in wanting to remain in her assisted living apartment. How do you think the situation should now be handled?

3. Some long-term care facilities have different sections for residents who are private pay and for residents on Medicaid. If Dorothy and Leo Hansen had been residents of such a facility, they would have been transferred to the Medicaid section of the facility when they could no longer pay their own way. From an ethical point of view, is this type of arrangement fair? Is it consistent with the concept of a right to health care?

4. The case of Dorothy and Leo Hansen is a case in which residents must leave a facility involuntarily and find placement elsewhere. Do you think that there are instances in which the involuntary discharge and relocation of residents is ethically justifiable?
   - Could the medical condition of a resident ever justify an involuntary discharge?
   - Could the behavior of a resident towards other residents or towards staff ever justify an involuntary discharge?
   - Does nonpayment of fees ever justify an involuntary discharge?
   To what ethical principles would you appeal to justify your responses?

5. How would you answer the question: "In view of the contributions the elderly have made to the society we now enjoy, what kind and quality of care do we owe them?"

NOTES

1. Robert L. Schneider, *The Relocation and Transfer of Older Persons When Decision-Making Combines with Ethics* (Washington, DC: American Association of Homes and Services for the Aging, 1994).
2. Joint Commission on Accreditation of Healthcare Organizations, 2002-2003 *Standards for Long Term Care* (Oakbrook Terrace, IL: Joint Commission Resources, 2002).
3. Loren E. Lomasky, "Letter of the Law: Eviction from Homes" in Rosalie A. Kane and Arthur L. Caplan (eds.), *Everyday Ethics Resolving Dilemmas in Nursing Home Life* (New York: Springer, 1990).
4. Robert L. Schneider, *The Admissions Process: Nursing Homes and Ethical Issues* (Washington, DC: American Association of Homes and Services for the Aging, 1994).
5. Allen Buchanan, "Health-Care Delivery and Resource Allocation," section "Rights to Health Care" in Robert M. Veatch (ed.), *Medical Ethics* (Boston: Jones and Bartlett, 1989).
6. Ronald Munson (ed.), *Intervention and Reflection Basic Issues in Medical Ethics*, 3rd ed. (Belmont, CA: Wadsworth, 1988), Part IV.9.

FOR FURTHER STUDY

- Lawrence R. Leonard, "The Ties that Bind: Life Care Contracts and Nursing Homes" in Marshall B. Kapp, Harvey E. Pies, and A. Edward Doudera, *Legal and Ethical Aspects of Health Care For the Elderly* (Ann Arbor, MI: Health Administration Press, 1985).

- Norman Daniels, *Am I My Parents' Keeper? An Essay on Justice Between the Young and the Old* (New York: Oxford, 1988).

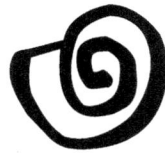

Chapter 4

Autonomy and Resident Rights

One of the difficulties a new resident can encounter in moving into a long-term care facility is the transition from living in a private home to living in an institutional setting. This setting involves learning to live within the context of a fairly large group of people who are strangers, both the other residents of the facility and staff members. It involves learning to live in an environment controlled by other people, namely, the facility's staff. It involves adjusting to predetermined daily schedules, and conforming to predetermined rules and regulations.

Studies indicate that "everyday events—not the dramatic medical decisions such as terminating life-sustaining treatment—comprise the majority of residents' concerns about autonomy." (1) Residents "want more control over day-to-day aspects of their lives and care, including their personal space, home or room, and day-to-day lifestyle." (2) Indeed, "as the baby boom generation ages and enters the long-term-care system, it is likely that their autonomy goals will be higher than those expressed by current cohorts." (2)

This chapter covers:
* *various dimensions of a resident's right to privacy;*
* *the movement to allow residents the right of choice in the activities of daily living;*
* *the relation of these rights to the ethical principle of autonomy.*

CASE STUDY
Roberta Boyle, now 78, had a very successful career as an attorney until she retired at the age of 72. She has never married, and has lived alone in her own home for most of her adult life. She is still very sharp mentally, but has developed severe back problems which make it difficult for her even to walk around her home. She could undergo back surgery, but she doesn't want to take the risks and face the long recovery period. Rather, she decides to try residency in the community's care center, where she will get assistance with daily living needs.

Roberta expected there to be adjustments when she moved into the Chelsea Care Facility. However, she did not expect to be "treated like a child."

Roberta wanted a private room, but only doubles are currently available. It is an adjustment in itself for Roberta to share a bedroom with another person who is a complete stranger. Roberta notices that the room door is always left open, and that staff seems to come into the room at will. She feels a lack of privacy when getting dressed and undressed, and when friends call her on the telephone. To make matters worse, one day a nurse came into the room and announced, right in front of Roberta's roommate, that she had a suppository to give to Roberta. Roberta found this quite embarrassing.

Then there is the daily routine. While she was living at home, Roberta used to stay up until midnight or 1:00 A.M. watching movies on television, then sleep until about 7:30 A.M. In the Chelsea Care Facility, it is "lights out" for everyone at 10:00 P.M. A nursing assistant comes around promptly at 6:00 A.M. to awaken Roberta and won't leave until Roberta has gotten out of bed and started to get dressed. Then Roberta has to wait until 7:30 A.M. before she can go to the dining room for breakfast. Since she is still capable of dressing herself, Roberta doesn't understand why she can't use her own alarm clock and choose the time to get up to be ready for breakfast.

There are some other things Roberta dislikes about living in the Chelsea Care Facility. She has been scheduled for a bath once a week on Tuesday morning. At home, Roberta had taken a bath several times a week, always in the evening. Then on Wednesday afternoons a church group from within the community has bingo for the residents of the facility. Roberta hates bingo, and would rather spend her time reading the latest issue of *Time* magazine. She has told this to the staff, but every week they still nag her to socialize with the other residents by playing bingo.

The staff also insists on keeping Roberta's blood pressure medication and being the ones to give her the pills daily. Roberta has been taking this medication for twenty years and administering it herself, and she doesn't see why she can't continue to do so now. In fact, she can't even keep a bottle of aspirin in her room. The staff tells her that the regulations of the facility require staff to control all medications. Roberta begins to wonder just what rights residents of long-term care facilities have!

The Right to Privacy

In its *Resident's Bill of Rights,* a long-term care facility may affirm a right to privacy:

> You have the right to every consideration of your privacy as it relates to your social, religious, and psychological well being and in your medical care program. Care discussion, consultation, examination, and treatment are confidential and will be conducted discretely.

> You have the right to send and receive your personal mail unopened, and have access to a telephone to make and receive calls with privacy. (3)

The right to privacy is grounded in the ethical principle of autonomy, for "respect for privacy is...one of the ways in which we symbolize our acknowledgment that the person is an autonomous agent who is in control of her life." (4) However, the case of Roberta Boyle illustrates difficulties that commonly occur in long-term care facilities in putting the commitment to residents' privacy into practice.

A home defines a private space for an individual. When an individual moves into a long-term care facility, his room becomes his "home." In making this move, the resident must divest himself of many possessions acquired throughout a lifetime. The resident's room will contain the few cherished possessions that he is able to bring with him and which help define his individuality. (4)

The number of private rooms in a long-term care facility is usually limited. When a resident has to share a room, as is the case with Roberta, even the sense of having her own private space is diminished.

Double rooms often have only a curtain suspended between the two beds. The privacy provided by pulling such a curtain is limited. Sounds and smells are not contained, and movement can be seen. When doors to resident rooms are left open, staff, other residents, and visitors can observe the residents from the hallway. Pulling a curtain across in a double room provides little privacy for residents living on the hallway side of the room. (4) Thus Roberta legitimately complains of feeling a lack of privacy when getting dresssed and undressed and when talking on the telephone.

The aforementioned *Resident's Bill of Rights* indicates that "care discussion, consultation, examination, and treatment are confidential and will be conducted discretely." A nurse openly stating Roberta's need for a suppository in front of her roommate violated Roberta's privacy regarding personal care needs. Even worse than staff discussing a resident's personal care needs indiscreetly are cases in which personal care is given in public areas of the facility:

> A somewhat different issue of bodily privacy was the staff's practice of routinely performing medical procedures such as cleaning leg ulcers, and changing IV bottles and feeding tubes in public areas such as the TV lounge. In fact, most procedures (excluding naso-gastric tubes) were done wherever the patients were when the staff found them. (4)

Roberta noted that staff comes into residents' room at will. Such staff intrusions can be embarrassing to residents and violate their bodily privacy. The following incident illustrates this point:

> One night I was putting her (Ms. Owen) back (into bed from the bathroom), and I was halfway getting her into bed. Her back end was sticking out, and (a male aide) came in the door. ...She just did a real quick turn around with her head, and she said, "Oh, get out of here!" I went and stood in front of her to kind of cover her up. (4)

Privacy has a psychological as well as a physical dimension. It sometimes involves having a place and a time to be alone. Roberta is in a double room, and other parts of the facility, such as lounges and even a chapel, are communal areas where others can come at will. (4) Staff even nags Roberta to socialize with other residents of the facility by playing bingo rather than spending time reading a news magazine by herself.

Privacy has a number of different dimensions. It involves privacy of space, privacy for one's body and personal care needs, privacy of communication, and the psychological privacy of being alone. (4) Some of the violations of residents' privacy noted above, such as staff walking into residents' rooms unannounced or performing medical procedures in public areas of the facility, can be addressed through training and sensitizing staff. Other problems, such as the lack of privacy inherent in the structure of double rooms and the lack of places where mentally competent residents can spend time alone, challenge us to think about the very design of long-term care facilities.

Schedules, Regulations, and the Right of Choice

Roberta Boyle was a successful professional woman who had managed on her own throughout her life. Yet when she entered a care facility, she found that other people now controlled much of her daily life. She is told when to go to bed and when to get up. Meal times are set for her. Others determine when and how many times she takes a bath. There are even pressures exerted on her regarding the kinds of leisure activities in which she engages. She must abide by regulations others have set regarding the administration of medication and what she can keep in her room.

It might be argued that, in voluntarily entering a long-term care facility, Roberta agreed (at least implicitly) to accept the rules and regulations that govern life in the facility. Because of her consent, she has a duty to comply without complaint. (1) On this view, it is older adults who are "expected to adapt to the systems." (2) Contrasting with this view is the movement which advocates changing environments to meet the needs and preferences of older clients (2) and "flexibility in the way that rules and procedures are applied to residents." (2)

For example, Roberta is forced to get up at 6:00 A.M. and to have breakfast at 7:30 A.M. Some older adults may be accustomed to sleeping later in the morning, or to having just a cup of coffee in the morning rather than a full breakfast. (1) To accommodate these personal preferences, a facility might have a continental breakfast available in a lounge area for two or three hours every morning.

Studies indicate that such arrangements will likely have a positive impact on the morale of residents:

> Making their own decisions about activities of daily living has been identified as one of the strongest influences on the morale of elderly nursing home residents... Scores on Chang's Situational Control of Daily Activities (SCDA) Scale... showed that of the eight areas of daily activity, grooming and eating were seen by most residents as the areas of their daily lives where they had the least control... If these findings are reliable, then freedom to make autonomous decisions about dining may strongly influence morale of elderly nursing home residents.

> More important, perhaps, Ryden...found that perceived situational control was the only variable that had a significant direct effect on the morale of residents on skilled care. According to Ryden, the greater the functional dependency, the less sense of control and the lower morale score. These results suggest to Ryden that the morale of competent residents could improve through interventions designed to increase their perception of situational control. (1)

For some time a *medical* model was prevalent in long-term care. Such a model "defines role relationships in which healthcare providers tell patients what to do rather than helping them to express and implement their own preferences." (2) On this model, "patients are expected to follow orders, not act independently." (2) In contrast, it is now being suggested that "nursing homes could learn a great deal from the hospitality industry about providing rooms, meals, and similar services." (2)

Autonomy, or self-determination, is a value that is much emphasized in contemporary health care ethics. One ethicist has proposed that the "principle of respect for autonomy...implies *individualized care* in the nursing home setting; it suggests that the provision of care, within limits, should follow the tracks set by the resident's autonomous choices..." (1)

Under the leadership of administrator Eric Haider, the Crestview Nursing Home in Bethany, Missouri, is one long-term care facility that has attempted to put this philosophy into practice. (5) Haider's personal experiences working in long-term care led him to focus on what the resident himself or herself wants:

> I was trying to get this lady dressed. I told her I'd do it my way...I was an 18-year-old kid. What was my experience with her garments? I was trying to prove that I was right, but who was I to tell her how to dress? (5)

> In one nursing home, I saw an aide giving an old lady a hug, telling her she loved her, that this was her home....Then the lady asked for something to eat and the aide told her no, that she'd have to wait until lunch time. Either this is their home or it isn't. Would you have to wait at home? Right then I thought, either quit lying to them or make it their home. (5)

At Haider's Crestview Nursing Home, "the new lobby looks much like a resort hotel, complete with waterfall and comfortable furniture." (5) Residents "decide what to eat and when, when to get up and what they want to do." (5) Meal times have been abolished, "replaced by continuous buffets which allow residents to eat whenever they want." (5) Many choices are offered to residents: "choice of fried chicken, sauerkraut and tomatoes, salad bar, liver and onions and much more for one day's lunch; choice of carpet or linoleum, drapes or blinds, wallpaper or paint, refrigerator or microwave, and decorations for each room." (5) One resident's room is "filled with American Indian hangings, a CD player and more than 100 CDs." (5)

It is important to note that this changed environment has resulted in better health for the residents. Hospital visits have been cut by 50 percent, the use of protective undergarments has been cut drastically, and the use of medication has declined sharply. (5)

Crestview Nursing Home received a standing ovation from state nursing home surveyors at a recognition dinner as well as a perfect score on a state inspection. It has been recognized in a resolution from the Missouri House of Representatives, and the Missouri Division of Aging wants to use it as a model home. (5)

FOR GROUP DISCUSSION

1. The standards for long-term care developed by the Joint Commission on Accreditation of Healthcare Organizations (JCAHO) affirm "the resident has a right to privacy, safety, and security." [RI.2.3] Specifically, a facility should support the resident's right to privacy by providing "visual and auditory privacy (for example, during visits, conversations, treatment and care procedures, and telephone calls)" and "privacy of written and oral communication." [Intent of RI.2.3] (6)

   If you are connected with a long-term care facility, examine the facility's bill of rights for residents (or a comparable document). What does it say about privacy for residents? Can you think of examples where the stipulations about privacy have been concretely put into practice? Can you think of any ways in which the privacy stipulations have been violated? Do you think any changes in the content of the document are in order with respect to residents' privacy? (If you are not connected with a long-term care facility, you might obtain the residents' bill of rights from several facilities and examine them.)

2. If you are connected with a long-term care facility, make a list of the rules and regulations, both written and informal, which govern daily life in the facility. Are prospective residents adequately informed of these rules and regulations during the admissions process? Looking at the list critically, do you think that any rules and regulations should be revised? Consistent with the ethical principle of autonomy, what role should residents themselves have in determining the rules and regulations governing daily life in the facility?

3. If you are connected with a long-term care facility, describe the "schedule" followed by a mentally competent resident for one week. Can you think of ways in which greater flexibility and choice might be introduced into the daily living of such residents? If you are a staff member of a long-term care facility who provides hands-on care for residents, how important do you find an established routine and schedule in getting your work done?

4. Imagine that you yourself are still mentally competent and have to move into a long-term care facility because of your physical care needs. List the five activities for which you would consider it most important to retain personal choice. If you are connected with a long-term care facility, consider whether you would be able to have those choices within the context of your facility.

5. It has been suggested that long-term care facilities might learn something about the provision of services from the hospitality industry. If you are a staff member in a long-term care facility, how do you feel about this suggestion?

6. The case of Roberta Boyle at the beginning of this chapter represents mentally competent residents who are capable of autonomous choices. However, the long-term care setting overall is more complex than this. Long-term care facilities typically include residents with cognitive impairments in varying degrees. Such residents need a structured environment. (4) A facility's

regulations and routines may have been "designed primarily for the more physically and mentally impaired" residents. (4) This may be the case, for example, with the rule which prohibits Roberta from even keeping a bottle of aspirin in her room. How can a long-term care facility develop an environment that allows residents with varying levels of ability to determine the course of their own lives?

7. Do you think that a list of "residents' responsibilities" should go along with a list of "residents' rights"? If so, what do you think should be included in the list of responsibilities?

8. In your facility you employ both male and female CNAs (certified nursing assistants) of various racial and ethnic backgrounds (Caucasian, Hispanic, African-American). The staffing situation is very tight.

   • Suppose that a female resident indicates to you that she wishes her personal care needs (including toileting and bathing) to be taken care of only by a female CNA. Should you honor her choice in assigning staff?

   • Suppose that a male resident makes it very clear that he does not want to be cared for by an African-American or Hispanic, and that he repeatedly makes derogatory remarks about them. Should you honor his choice in assigning staff?

   • While there is an emphasis on the staff of long-term care facilities learning to cater to the preferences of residents, do you think there are situations in which the lifestyle choice of a resident should not be honored?

NOTES

1. Rosalie A. Kane and Arthur L. Caplan (eds.), *Everyday Ethics Resolving Dilemmas in Nursing Home Life* (New York: Springer, 1990).
2. Brian L. Hofland and Debra David, "Autonomy and Long-Term-Care Practice: Conclusions and Next Steps," *Generations* 92 Suppl. (1990): 91-94.
3. *Resident's Bill of Rights*, Stonehill Care Center, Dubuque, Iowa (1999).
4. Charles W. Lidz, Lynn Fischer, and Robert M. Arnold, *The Erosion of Autonomy in Long-Term Care* (New York: Oxford University Press, 1992).
5. Julie Belschner, "A place to enjoy life—home caters to residents," *St. Joseph News-Press*, February 20, 2000.
6. Joint Commission on Accreditation of Healthcare Organizations, 2002-2003 *Standards for Long Term Care* (Oakbrook Terrace, IL: Joint Commission Resources, 2002).

FOR FURTHER STUDY

• "Resident Privacy—Mrs. Gardner" in Diane E. Hoffmann, Philip Boyle, and Steven A. Levenson, *Handbook for Nursing Home Ethics Committees* (Washington, DC: American Association of Homes and Services for the Aging, 1995).

- "If You Let Them They'd Stay in Bed All Morning: The Tyranny of Regulation in Nursing Home Life," "Thought for Food: Nursing Home Meals" and "Phone Privileges" in Rosalie A. Kane and Arthur L. Caplan (eds.), *Everyday Ethics Resolving Dilemmas in Nursing Home Life* (New York: Springer, 1990).

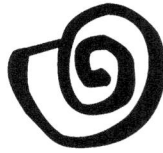

Chapter 5

Everyday Dilemmas for Staff and Residents

Health care ethics has come to be associated with critical life-and-death decisions. Should antibiotics be given to a resident with end stage Alzheimer's disease who has developed pneumonia? Should tube feeding be withdrawn from a resident in a persistent vegetative state? Can assisted suicide ever be ethically justifiable?

Ethics, however, pertains to all facets of life. One of the challenges of ethics education is to sensitize health care providers to the ethical dimensions of seemingly mundane situations. This chapter will examine, from an ethical perspective, five issues commonly encountered in daily living in a long-term care facility.

Specifically, this chapter covers:
* *the allocation of private rooms in a long-term care facility;*
* *the assignment of roommates;*
* *negotiating acceptable levels of risk taking with residents;*
* *the use of common spaces in a long-term care facility;*
* *staff receiving gifts from residents.*

CASE STUDY
Anita Richards, the administrator of the Montrose Care Center, wishes that the facility had been built with all private rooms. If it had been, her life as an administrator would be much less stressful. But, as things stand, only fifteen of the seventy-five rooms in the facility are singles. She must ultimately make the decision about which residents get to have private rooms and which ones must share doubles-which has its own set of problems with matching compatible roommates!

One private room has just become available due to the death of a long-time resident. Anita has narrowed down the potential candidates for moving into this room to three persons.

One candidate is Genevieve Collins, who has been a resident at the Montrose Care Center for two years. Genevieve is currently in a double room with a woman who suffers from dementia. She doesn't talk much with Genevieve or with anyone else. She is basically harmless, but she does become agitated when Genevieve turns on the small television set or radio in her section of the room. Thus Genevieve doesn't listen to them nearly as much as she would like to do. Genevieve has been on the facility's waiting list for a private room since she was admitted to the Montrose Care Center, and she is now at the top of the waiting list.

A second candidate is Frank Vosberg. Frank is currently in a double room, and has had four roommates in the last year, all of whom have asked to be transferred to another double room. Frank spent his life as a farmer, and he remains very strong physically. His major functional disability is dementia, which causes him to exhibit behavior disturbing to his roommates. He rummages through the dresser drawers of his roommates, taking items of clothing or toiletries that he then uses himself. Worst of all, when Frank gets up at night to go to the bathroom, he sometimes forgets which bed in the room belongs to him. He goes to his roommate's bed, and thinking that the roommate is a stranger who is in his bed, lifts the person out of the bed and puts him on the floor. Staff is concerned that Frank may some day injure a resident by this behavior.

A third candidate is John Baker, a new resident who will be admitted from the hospital in just a few days. John is terminally ill, and will be part of the facility's hospice program. He is expected to die within three months.

Anita struggles with the question of who should be placed in the single room.

Allocating the Scarce Resource of Private Rooms

Long-term care facilities, as they are currently built, typically do not have enough private rooms to accommodate all the residents who would like to have one. Thus, somewhat analogous to transplant organs, private rooms fall into the category of a scarce health care resource. Concomitantly, principles must be developed to govern the fair allocation of them.

One proposed set of criteria establishes the following priorities.

- First and foremost, the welfare of the entire community of residents should be taken into account. Specifically, harm to other residents should be avoided. Thus, first priority for placement in private rooms should be given, for example, to residents needing isolation to prevent the spread of an infectious disease and to residents who are assaultive. (1)

- Second, priority should be given to residents who are dying. This is to be done out of deference "to the privacy claim of dying residents and their families" and in order "to shelter roommates from having another person (usually a stranger) die within their social interpersonal distance zone." (1)

- Third, resort should be made to a waiting list. Priority should be given on the waiting list to long-staying residents over short-staying residents (i.e., residents admitted for rehabilitation, convalescence, terminal care, or caregiver respite). Priority should be given to the long-staying residents for the reason that the facility is their *home*, not a temporary, transitional situation. (1)

If the administrator of Montrose Care Center used this set of criteria, who would be placed in the private room that has become available? Frank Vosberg would have first priority for the private room. This is because his assaultive behavior towards his roommates, in taking them out of bed and putting them on the floor, has the potential to harm them.

When another private room becomes available, these criteria would determine that it should go to John Baker. Although he is a new admission, he is dying.

If a third private room becomes available, it should go to Genevieve Collins. This is because she is a long-term resident who is at the top of the waiting list.

The authors of the above set of criteria introduce an additional factor into the third priority level, namely, the financial resources of residents. They propose that long-staying residents who are private pay should have priority over long-staying residents who cannot pay their own way and are dependent on governmental assistance. Similarly, if one finally reaches the level of short-staying residents, it is again claimed that those who are private pay should have priority over those who are not. (1) The rationale behind this proposal is that

> ...equal access to equal-quality housing is not a right that our society recognizes. People who have more money can and do purchase more spacious or better appointed houses. ...wealthier long-term residents may be allowed to have priority for the costlier single rooms. (1)

This stipulation is likely to provoke discussion and some controversy. Consider, for example, the case of Genevieve Collins. Montrose Care Center is her home, and having a private room is likely to bring a distinct improvement in the quality of her living situation. Suppose, however, that she is one of those residents who has exhausted her own financial resources paying for her long-term care and is now on a governmental assistance program. From an ethical point of view, is it fair to deny her an improvement in the quality of her life on financial grounds? More basically, should the best quality living situation in a long-term care facility be a luxury item available only to those who can afford it?

CASE STUDY

Although it is not one of the more pleasant aspects of her job as administrator of the Montrose Care Center, Anita Richards must also make hard decisions about the assignment of roommates.

Two months ago John and Mary Bishop moved into the facility. Since they had been married for fifty-two years, they assumed they would have a room together. However, no double room was available at the time, and they were split up into different double rooms.

Recently, the roommate of Marsha Walker and the roommate of Sarah Fahey have died. John Bishop goes to see Anita Richards to suggest that Marsha and Sarah could now share a room, thus making a double room available for him and his wife to share.

However, when Anita approaches Marsha about sharing a room with Sarah, Marsha vigorously objects. Marsha points out that Sarah is "out of it mentally" and that she has a reputation for getting into the personal belongings of her roommates. Sarah has damaged food and gifts that family members have brought to her roommates. Marsha further tells Anita that she has now been a resident at the Montrose Care Center for five years, all of which have been spent in the room she currently occupies. She makes it clear that she should have a say in who moves into "her room."

Anita knows that, if she transfers Sarah into Marsha's room against Marsha's wishes, there is likely to be serious conflict between them. On the other hand, Anita sympathizes with the plight of John and Mary Bishop. She struggles with the dilemma of who should be roommates for nearly a week before making a decision.

Assigning Roommates

Determining roommates is perhaps one of the most challenging dilemmas pertaining to day-to-day living in a long-term care facility. Often complete strangers are suddenly thrown together, without choice, and expected to get along. Limited availability of rooms within a facility may necessitate placing a mentally alert resident with someone suffering from dementia, as happened to Genevieve Collins at the Montrose Care Center and may happen to Marsha Walker.

What principles can be used to make these difficult decisions? We will consider three different approaches, and their concrete implications for the case at hand.

The first approach is similar in form and content to that used for making allocation decisions about private rooms. It involves using a list of priorities of the following sort:

- Priority for sharing a room should first be given to married couples. This is because of the societal recognition given to the state of marriage. (1)

- Second, roommates should be determined according to the preferences of the residents themselves. In this regard, long-staying residents who are able to pay their own way should be given first pick of roommates. The choice of roommates falls secondly to long-staying residents who are not able to pay their own way; thirdly, to short-staying residents who are able to pay; and fourthly, to short-staying residents who are not able to pay. (1)

Using these criteria, the fact that John and Mary Bishop are married would be the determining factor in assigning rooms. At first glance, it seems plausible to try to preserve the value of a long-standing marital relationship within a facility, unless separation is absolutely necessary for the level of care one of the partners requires. But this decision would also mean that Marsha and Sarah could be forced to share a room together, so that a double room could be made available to the Bishops. Intuitively, is there a feeling that Marsha's rights are being violated in having a roommate forced on her whom she clearly does not want? Further, does not Marsha's length of stay at the facility give her some prerogatives over newcomers to the facility?

A different approach comes out of the tradition of an ethics of justice. It involves evaluating ethical dilemmas in terms of a hierarchy of rights. (2) In this approach, "the rights of each individual are weighed and tallied, and whoever is seen as having the most rights or the most important rights is deemed the one whose demands are to be fulfilled over those of the others, who have less of a right." (2) In the case at hand, John and Mary Bishop can assert a right to be together based on their marital relationship. Marsha Walker, on the other hand, can assert a right to privacy. In particular, Marsha can claim a right to be free of roommates (such as Sarah Fahey) who will not respect her personal property. But how does one weigh these competing rights? As seen in the previous chapter, a right to privacy is an important one for residents of long-term care facilities. In its own way, is not privacy just as important to Marsha as their marital relationship is to John and Mary?

A third way of approaching this dilemma comes from the feminist ethics of care. This ethical theory focuses on the network of relationships involved in a situation:

> It is no longer a matter of looking at each participant in the conflict individually and evaluating his or her rights, separated from the rights of the rest of the people involved. Instead, the situation as a whole is evaluated, taking not just individual rights but other factors into account. What is sought is a solution, usually much more complex and multifaceted than that which an ethics of justice provides, one that takes each individual's needs into account and tries to satisfy each one as best it can. (2)

The ethics of care would challenge the administrator of the Montrose Care Center to think creatively about possible solutions to the roommate problem that would satisfy the needs of all the players in this situation. Given her problem with dementia and its accompanying disruptive behavior, would it be best for Sarah to be placed in a private room as soon as one becomes available? Then John and Mary Bishop could move into her double room, and Marsha Walker could be consulted about her preferences for a new roommate. Or would Sarah be compatible with Mary Bishop's current roommate, so that Mary could move into Sarah's room with her husband? Or again, would Marsha find Mary's current roommate acceptable as her new roommate, so that John could share Mary's current room? These solutions have the advantage of respecting Marsha Walker's preferences for a roommate while still finding a way for John and Mary Bishop to live together as husband and wife.

CASE STUDY

Don Carter, 77, has been living alone for the past two years since the death of his wife. His daughter, who checks on him daily, has noticed that he has become increasingly forgetful over the past year. Don forgets to turn off lights. After being on blood pressure medication for some twenty years, he now no longer remembers to take it daily. Sometimes he misplaces money at home. However, the worst incident occurred three months ago when Don was driving home from a nearby grocery store. He got lost, and drove around for over an hour before he found his way home. Don's doctor believes that this behavior likely represents early stage dementia.

Don agrees to move into a residential unit of the Sunset Park Home. He has given up his own car, but a city bus stops right in front of the facility. Don starts taking the bus to the local senior center so that he can continue to play euchre with his old friends several afternoons a week.

Staff at the Sunset Park Home has mixed feelings about Don's excursions. On the one hand, they see the trips to the senior center as having distinct benefits for him mentally and psychologically. Unlike many residents of Sunset Park, Don has something he can look forward to doing. Playing euchre with old friends provides some degree of mental stimulation for him as well as ongoing socialization.

On the other hand, staff fears that Don may suffer a bout of forgetfulness while on one of these excursions. They fear that he will get off at the wrong stop, start walking, and get totally lost. In fact, there was recently a story in the newspaper about a man who wandered off from a long-term care facility and was attacked and beaten up. Staff wouldn't want this to happen to Don. They wonder if they should put a stop to Don's excursions for his own good.

Allowing Residents to Take Risks

This is a classic case of a conflict between staff concerns over the safety of a resident and a resident's self-determination of the activities of his or her own life. It has been pointed out that

> ...the prevailing philosophical paradigm underlying residential services for the elderly has been one emphasizing protection of the client from any anticipated potential harm. This approach to providing services is predicated on the fundamental ethical principles of beneficence, or doing good for others, and nonmaleficence (Primum non nocere, "First, Do No Harm.") These traditionally have been the guiding precepts of health and human services professions. (3)

The focus on protecting residents from harm has been reinforced by concerns over legal liability in a very litigious society. (3, 4)

However, a paradigm shift has recently been taking place. This paradigm shift, which is evident in assisted living (3) but is also applicable to the context of long-term care, involves a commitment on the part of service providers to individual autonomy. (3) Under this model, "particular clients are presumed to be adults who are capable of formulating, expressing, and acting upon their own values and preferences regarding both major life decisions and smaller, but nonetheless important, choices arising in everyday life." (3)

Using this new paradigm, it has been suggested that the moral responsibility of health care providers to prevent harm from coming to residents can be reconciled with individual autonomy through a process called "negotiated risk." (3) This process involves informing the competent resident of the potential harm involved in his current behavior, proposing and exploring various alternative courses of action which could be taken, and then allowing the resident to choose a course of action to respond to the problem. The resident's choice could involve acceptance of certain risks of injury. (3) From a staff point of view, the process of negotiated risk involves thinking creatively about alternative, and perhaps non-traditional, ways of dealing with a problem.

The following is an example of the process of negotiated risk:

> Diane D is an insulin-dependent diabetic, with orders from her physician for adherence to an American Diabetes Association diet. However, she likes sweets and frequently asks staff for desserts after meals. On occasion,

staff have refused her request, and she has taken desserts from her table-mates. She says that she does not like diabetic desserts.

Diane wishes to continue to eat desserts. If she continues to do so, she could elevate her blood sugar to a level that could place her at an extreme health risk. Alternatives to minimize the risk can include: Staff can offer Diane more of a variety of diabetic desserts, including those that the individual says she would prefer; Diane agrees not to request non-diabetic desserts (the staff will not give her non-diabetic desserts); Diane is informed of the health risks involved in eating desserts, and chooses for herself if she wants to continue to eat desserts.

A final agreement, reached between Diane and the caregiver, will have the food services staff talk to Diane to find out which diabetic desserts she would be most likely to enjoy, and will serve those desserts to Diane. Diane agrees to discuss all possible risks with her physician and to sign an agreement that she understands all consequences of eating desserts. She will then choose whether she prefers to eat the diabetic desserts, regular desserts, or no desserts at all.

Diane liked one diabetic dessert that the staff fixed for her, and ate this dessert most of the time. Occasionally she ate a non-diabetic dessert, but was able to keep her blood sugar level under control. (3)

How might the process of negotiated risk apply to the case of Don Carter? At present, Don decides on his own to take the city bus to the senior center whenever he wishes to do so. However, because of his occasional forgetful behavior, it is possible that he could get off at the wrong stop and start wandering around, getting lost. If this happens, he might also be put in the position of being vulnerable to crime. These are the risks involved in his behavior.

Don wants to continue going to the senior center to play euchre with friends, and staff agrees that this is a beneficial thing for him to do. Alternatives to minimize the risk include at least the following options:

- Don continues to take the bus but agrees to inform staff at the facility when he plans to go to the senior center and of his expected time of return to the facility. At the appropriate time, staff make a point of checking that Don has in fact returned.

- Don continues to take the bus but agrees to inform staff at the facility when he plans to go to the senior center and to invest in a cellular telephone to carry with him on these excursions. The telephone will allow him to call the facility immediately in the event that he gets lost. Staff will check that Don has the telephone with him before he leaves the facility.

- Arrangements are made to have Don's friends from the senior center provide transportation for him to and from the senior center. Don agrees to go to the senior center only when this transportation is available.

- Arrangements are made to have community volunteers who work at the facility provide transportation for Don to and from the senior center. Don agrees to go to the senior center only when these community volunteers are available as drivers.

Let us suppose that Don chooses the second alternative. This alternative carries a greater degree of risk than the third and fourth alternatives in that Don could still get lost. However, Don accepts this degree of risk in order to have the freedom to go to the senior center to play euchre whenever he wishes, something not necessarily allowed by the third and fourth options.

It must be recognized that there are challenges in putting this model into practice. In our case Don is still in the early stages of dementia, and it has been assumed that his decision-making powers are still intact. However, many residents of long-term care facilities suffer from a much greater degree of cognitive impairment, and family members and staff must learn how to maximize opportunities for decision making for such individuals. (3) Further, there will be some residents who are completely incapable of making decisions. In these cases, a proxy decision maker must assess what kind and degree of risks the individual would be willing to assume if able to make a decision. (3)

CASE STUDY

One of the problems the staff of the Heartland Care Center must deal with is smoking on the part of residents. The staff is generally in agreement that, ideally, Heartland Care Center should be a smoke-free environment. After all, Heartland Care Center is a facility dedicated to health care, and smoking has been proven to be unhealthful. However, there are some residents who have smoked for years and don't even want to try to give it up. The staff has decided that, out of respect for the autonomy of these residents, a place will be made available to accommodate smokers.

During the winter months, a particular lounge area is set aside for the smokers. When the weather is warm, the smokers are asked to go outdoors to smoke.

There is a very nice patio area in back of the building which has been built through donations made by a local church group expressly for this purpose. The smokers have naturally started to congregate in this area. However, non-smoking residents who want to sit outdoors on the patio complain that the smoke is bothering them.

The smokers feel that they are respecting the rights of the non-smokers by not smoking inside the building. They feel that the non-smokers should in turn respect their rights by allowing them to have the patio area in which to smoke. In fact, one smoker recently brought a sign to the patio that reads, "Hassling me about my smoking may be dangerous to your health."

The issue of who gets to use the patio is finally taken to the Residents' Council for resolution.

The Use of Common Spaces

The patio at the Heartland Care Center has been provided through donations made by a local church group expressly for this purpose. Undoubtedly, this group intended the patio to serve all the residents of the facility, not just a particular group. It was intended to be a "common space." Just what constitutes fairness in the use of such common spaces?

It is too strong to say that all residents should have access to a common space at all times. In general, it is accepted practice in our society that rooms can be reserved by an individual or a group for a particular activity for a particular time period. For example, some banks have rooms that can be reserved for meetings by various groups and organizations within the community. What constitutes unfairness is if a particular individual or group who is entitled to have access to a space is completely excluded from using it. For example, it would be unfair and discriminatory if, all things being equal, the East Side Kiwanis Club was allowed to use the bank's meeting room while the West Side Kiwanis Club was not.

Some find it disagreeable and annoying to be in close proximity to persons who are smoking. Because of allergies and diseases, some simply cannot physically tolerate smoking by other people. Some wish to avoid smokers because of the effects of second-hand smoke. For these reasons, some residents of the Heartland Care Center may claim that letting smokers congregate on the patio is de facto excluding them completely from using the patio area. Since the non-smokers are among the residents of the Heartland Care Center for whom the patio was intended, they could argue that it is unfair that the smokers be allowed to use the patio all the time.

A compromise solution might be to reserve use of the patio at certain hours for smokers and at other hours for non-smokers, with the smokers being provided with another outdoor area at the times they are unable to use the patio. This would be in accord with the accepted societal practice of reserving rooms. Or, if the patio area is large enough, the staff might designate "smoking" and "non-smoking" sections of the patio, just as there are smoking and non-smoking sections of many restaurants.

The smokers argue that they are respecting the rights of the non-smokers by not smoking inside the building, and thus that the non-smokers should in turn respect their rights by allowing them to have the patio area in which to smoke. However, this proposed division of territory ignores the fact that the patio is a common area of the facility that all residents are entitled to use at some time or other.

It might be pointed out that, when the weather does not permit use of the patio, one particular lounge within the facility is set aside for the smokers. Are not lounges intended to be common areas? And is this not dividing up territory within the facility between smokers and non-smokers?

If there is more than one lounge area within the facility and the smoking and non-smoking lounges are comparable, then it would seem that both smoking and non-smoking residents are being treated equally and fairly. There is, however, only one patio area available for the residents, so that the analogy breaks down.

Nevertheless, this argument suggests a modification to the principle that all residents should have access to a common area at some time or other. Perhaps considerations of justice and fairness are satisfied if comparable spaces are made available to different groups of residents.

CASE STUDY

Ever since she assumed the position of administrator of the Lutheran Home, Linda Johnson has emphasized to the staff the creation of a caring, home-like environment, and showing a personal interest in the residents. However, the efforts of staff to achieve these goals have had an unexpected consequence. A number of residents and their family members have given gifts to staff for "doing their job."

For example, the daughter of Mrs. Kane bought a scarf for a nurse to show appreciation for the special attention she gave to her mother when her mother was ill for a week with the flu and suffering bouts of incontinence. Mrs. Springer still crochets, and gave an item she had made to a CNA on her birthday. At Christmas time, the family of Mr. Caplan brought tins of homemade cookies to each of the staff working on the wing where their father resides.

One resident, Emma Brody, has confided to Linda Johnson that she feels badly that she can't give anything to her caregivers to show her appreciation for the attention they give her. This comment makes Linda Johnson wonder if all this gift giving is really a good thing. She decides to raise this issue for discussion at the next meeting of the facility's management team.

Gifts to Staff

Giving personal gifts in a workplace setting can be a way of treating an employee as a "person" and not just an entity to perform services. It can be a sign of respect as well as gratitude. It can help create a work environment where people feel that they are valued, which in turn contributes to job satisfaction.

On one level, it is a positive development that the staff at the Lutheran Home has achieved such a caring interpersonal relationship with residents and their family members that they naturally feel inclined to go beyond paying the residency fees and to give gifts to staff members. However, there are some hidden dangers in the practice of giving gifts in the long-term care context.

For one thing, adequate staffing is often a problem in long-term care facilities so that decisions must be made about the allocation of staff time among various residents. If a staff member has received a gift from a resident or his family, that staff member may feel somewhat indebted to that resident and, perhaps without consciously realizing it, tend to favor that resident over others in terms of priority for caregiving. In other words, the practice of staff receiving gifts has the potential to lead to unfair favoritism in the treatment of residents. (5)

Further, even if no favoritism occurs, residents who have not provided gifts to staff members may fear being slighted by staff or may think (however wrongly) that residents who give gifts will receive better treatment. Even the appearance or perception of favoritism is something to be avoided. (5)

Finally, residents differ in their ability to give gifts to staff, much as they might like to do this. (5) Some may be operating under financial constraints. Some may not have family available to help them provide gifts. Some may no longer be physically able even to make gifts—such as crocheted items—as they once used to do. Thus, the practice of residents giving gifts to staff may lead to those residents who cannot do so feeling inferior to the others.

For these reasons, a facility may wish to establish a blanket policy against staff accepting gifts from residents. Such a policy should be made known to residents and family members at the time of admission and to staff members at the time they are hired. It might also be reiterated periodically at staff meetings and in facility newsletters to residents and family members.

FOR GROUP DISCUSSION

1. Consider the dilemma faced by Anita Richards as administrator of the Montrose Care Center in having to decide which resident should be placed in the private room. If you had to decide among Genevieve Collins, Frank Vosberg, and John Baker, which one would you choose? How would you prioritize the remaining two residents? Very importantly, what factors are significant to you in making these decisions?

2. Consider the dilemma faced by Anita Richards as administrator of the Montrose Care Center in assigning roommates. If you were Anita, how would you handle the situation with John and Mary Bishop, Marsha Walker, and Sarah Fahey? Very importantly, what factors are significant to you in making your decision?

3. If you are connected with a long-term care facility, list the considerations which, as a matter of fact, are being used to make decisions about the allocation of private rooms and the assignment of roommates. Can any patterns be discerned? Does the facility have any written policies in place to guide these decisions? How do these policies compare with the principles and approaches outlined in the text?

4. Make a list of risks you are prepared to take in your own life. Is your risk taking comparable to allowing the residents of a long-term care facility to take risks? Or do you think there are important differences?

5. Within private homes, rooms like the kitchen, dining room, living room and family room are effectually "common spaces" for family members. Upon reflection, can you articulate any rules that, implicitly or explicitly, govern the use of these spaces by family members within your own home? Can any analogies be drawn for the use of common spaces in long-term care facilities?

6. Suppose that the family of a resident wished to share produce from their garden or farm with a facility. In this case, the gift would not go to particular staff members but to the facility as a whole. Is this an acceptable practice, or do you see any hidden dangers?

NOTES

1. "Intimate Strangers: Roommates in Nursing Homes" in Rosalie A. Kane and Arthur L. Caplan (eds.), *Everyday Ethics Resolving Dilemmas in Nursing Home Life* (New York: Springer, 1990).
2. "Till Death Us Do Part: Married Life in Nursing Homes" in Rosalie A. Kane and Arthur L. Caplan (eds.), *Everyday Ethics Resolving Dilemmas in Nursing Home Life* (New York: Springer, 1990).
3. Marshall B. Kapp and Keren Brown Wilson, "Assisted Living and Negotiated Risk: Reconciling Protection and Autonomy," *Journal of Ethics, Law, and Aging* 1/1 (1995): 5-13.
4. "Leaving Homes: Residents on Their Own Recognizance" in Rosalie A. Kane and Arthur L. Caplan (eds.), *Everyday Ethics Resolving Dilemmas in Nursing Home Life* (New York: Springer, 1990).
5. "Tips and Favors" in Rosalie A. Kane and Arthur L. Caplan (eds.), *Everyday Ethics Resolving Dilemmas in Nursing Home Life* (New York: Springer, 1990).

FOR FURTHER STUDY

• "The Chair and Other Public Space" and "Leaving Homes: Residents on Their Own Recognizance" in Rosalie A. Kane and Arthur L. Caplan, *Everyday Ethics Resolving Dilemmas in Nursing Home Life* (New York: Springer, 1990).

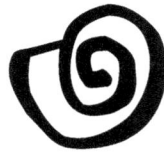

Chapter 6

Male-Female Relationships

Issues of male-female relationships and of human sexuality do not disappear when one enters the context of long-term care. Facilities may face decisions about elderly persons who are not married wishing to share living quarters. In some instances staff in long-term care facilities "have been asked to facilitate sexual activity" on the part of residents. (1) In some instances staff "have actually participated in or even initiated such activity" themselves. (1) Indeed, cases of residents' hiring prostitutes have been reported, "necessitating policy formulations based on both the facility's sponsorship or beliefs and the law." (1)

It is generally recognized in professional codes of ethics that persons providing health care should not engage in a sexual relationship with their clients. (1) This is especially important in the long-term care context because of "the inherently dependent status of residents." (1) However, other types of issues surrounding male-female relationships and sexuality on the part of residents have not received the same attention.

In our culture, the view of sexuality among older persons is primarily negative (2), and there seems to be an expectation that older people are, or ought to be, asexual. (3) However, "age itself abolishes neither the need nor the capacity for sexual activity...and many people enjoy a fulfilling sex life to the end of their lives." (3) Spouses may wish to continue a sexual relationship even though one or both of them have taken up residency in a long-term care facility. Nevertheless, "most institutions rigidly suppress sexuality in older residents," sometimes under pressure from children of nursing home residents. (4)

In addition to the issue of cohabitation, sexual relationships may be desired and established between two residents who are not married, somtimes even if a spouse is still living but residing outside the facility. Of particular concern have been sexual relationships involving residents suffering from dementia.

Staff of long-term care facilities may well see a range of sexual behaviors on the part of residents. It may include "companionship/courtship behaviors"; that is, "mutual displays of affection that are normally accepted in public, such as hand-holding, hugging, and kissing." (5) Some residents may display "self-stimulation behaviors," such as "masturbation, reading sexually explicit media materials, or public exposure." (5) Some residents may make "unwanted verbal and/or physical advances...toward other residents, staff or visitors"; for example, "passes, propositions, suggestive comments or gestures, grabbing or touching." (5) And some residents may engage in "sexually intimate behaviors generally reserved for private settings," such as "prolonged kissing, other forms of coupled stimulation, and sexual intercourse." (5)

This chapter covers:
- *cohabitation by couples who are not married;*
- *residents' rights with regard to sexual activity;*
- *sexual activity involving residents with dementia;*
- *when sexual activity involving residents may be appropriately curtailed by a facility.*

CASE STUDY

Rita Tucker, 79, and Tim Shannon, 81, both lost their spouses four years ago. They met at the community senior center, and became good friends. A year and a half ago, Tim invited Rita to move into the large home he had kept after the death of his wife. Contrary to the wishes of her children, Rita accepted his invitation. They both enjoyed each other's company, and Rita had often felt lonely in her apartment. She would also be able to save some money by giving up the apartment.

Rita is now becoming increasingly frail and Tim is having problems with walking because of severe arthritis. They both decide it is time to move into the residential floor of the care facility in their community, where meals and cleaning services will be provided as well as assistance with various daily needs. In this way they believe they can enjoy more the years remaining to them.

Tim and Rita make an appointment for an admissions interview at the Lake Park Home. Initially, all seems to go well. They tell the administrator, Alice Kramer, that they would like to share a room on the first floor residential unit of the home. It happens that a couple will be moved to the second floor at the end of the month because of their increased need for nursing care, creating a vacancy in the residential unit.

When Tim and Rita complete the admissions papers, Alice learns that they are not married. She is surprised by this, and doesn't know how to respond. Lake Park Home has never before been faced with a request by two unmarried people to live together in the facility as a married couple would. Alice allows them to complete the admissions papers, but tries to buy some time by telling them that processing the papers will take at least two weeks.

As soon as Tim Shannon and Rita Tucker leave her office, Alice Kramer calls the chair of the facility's ethics committee to arrange an ethics consult to discuss this unusual case.

Cohabitation

The type of case represented by Rita Tucker and Tim Shannon is likely to become more common in the future as individuals age who have had non-traditional ideas about marriage and sexuality throughout their lives. Should the cohabitation of persons who are not married be allowed in long-term care facilities?

Legally, Rita and Tim were perfectly free to maintain the relationship of unmarried persons that they had established within their own home. From a legal perspective, the burden of proof seems to lie with the facilities that wish to exclude a relationship of cohabitation from continuing into the long-term care setting. From an ethical point of view, it could be argued that the consciences of individuals regarding the practice of cohabitation should be respected by long-term care facilities. (1)

When the case of Rita and Tim is discussed by the ethics committee of Lake Park Home, a consideration that might be raised is the impact on other residents of allowing cohabitation within the facility. Some residents may well regard this arrangement as immoral. Rita and Tim may be socially ostracized by them, creating tensions in the daily living situation within the facility. Concomitantly, some residents may see the facility as condoning immoral behavior by allowing cohabitation, and wish to move to another facility. However, it is not clear that these considerations represent harms to residents that are serious enough to outweigh the legal freedom that Rita and Tim might claim to live together unmarried.

Suppose that, instead of seeking admission at a community facility like the Lake Park Home, Rita and Tim sought admission at the St. Francis Home. If a facility is religiously sponsored by a church (such as the Catholic Church) which has a clearly stated position against the ethical permissibility of cohabitation (6) , then the situation is different. It can be argued that it is part of the very mission of the facility to operate in accord with the principles of the church with which it is affiliated, and that practices not in accord with these principles can be prohibited. Nevertheless, as a matter of legal protection, such facilities should have a written policy excluding the cohabitation of unmarried persons and share that policy with prospective residents.

A long-term care facility may also receive admissions applications from couples who are gay or lesbian. If the administration of a facility would consider such couples living together in the facility to be problematic, a written policy should be formulated including the justification for the exclusion of such couples.

CASE STUDY
The case of Rita Tucker and Tim Shannon is not the first time that issues of male-female relationships have arisen at the Lake Park Home.

John and Mary Jane Brandt, both 75, have been married for fifty-two years. They moved into the residential unit of the Lake Park Home just four months ago. John suffers from some paralysis in one of his arms due to a stroke. Mary Jane's eyesight has become progressively worse, and she has almost reached the stage of being considered legally blind. In spite of these physical impairments, both remain active and take part in almost all the facility's cultural and social activities. On occasion, they still enjoy having sex.

One evening, three weeks after John and Mary Jane moved into the Lake Park Home, an unfortunate incident occurred. While they were having sex in their room, a nurse walked in to administer the medication they take before going to bed. The nurse reported their activity to the facility's administrator as inappropriate behavior that ought to be monitored. John, on the other hand, complained at the residents' council meeting about a lack of privacy in the facility.

Sexual Activity Between Spouses

In the case of John and Mary Jane Brandt, a nurse at the Lake Park Home judges their engagement in sexual relations to be "inappropriate behavior that ought to be monitored" and reports it to the facility's administrator. But should it be viewed as "inappropriate behavior"? After all, John and Mary Jane have been married for fifty-two years, and it is not regarded as ethically problematic for married persons to have a sexual relationship. If John and Mary Jane were still able to live at home, there would be no question about their right to engage in a sexual relationship. Is there something about the context of a long-term care facility that makes such a sexual relationship inappropriate?

The point might be raised that a long-term care facility is one type of health care facility and, as such, that it falls within the scope of the facility's role to discourage or prevent sexual activity that might harm a resident physically or psychologically. (2) However, we have no reason to think that this consideration applies to the case of John and Mary Jane. Indeed, it has been argued that "facilitating the expression of sexuality among elderly residents may result in a higher quality of life" (2):

> Butler and Lewis suggest that sexual orgasm relieves anxiety and contributes to the general well-being of the elderly individual. Kassel states that "sex is an opportunity for good clean entertainment that provides laughter and joy in the heart and the intimate giving of one person to the other." Sexual relationships could provide love, intimacy, and closeness, as well as physical stimulation—all of which could serve as motivating factors for continued or improved quality of life. (2)

In previous chapters we have explored resident autonomy and the issue of resident rights. We have seen that the current emphasis is on promoting the opportunities of residents to continue to control the course of their own lives as much as possible. Those who have qualms about the moral permissibility of cohabitation would not question that married persons have a right to sexual relations with each other. Thus it could be argued that, consistent with resident autonomy, the facility should permit residents like John and Mary Jane to continue their sexual relationship if they so choose, and provide an appropriate environment for it.

What remains an issue in the case of John and Mary Jane is that of staff behavior. Apparently, the nurse walked into John and Mary Jane's room unannounced to give them their medication. We can even wonder if the nurse took it upon himself or herself to open a closed door without knocking. The nurse's behavior can be construed as a violation of residents' right to privacy. If adequate privacy for sexual relations cannot be assured for John and Mary Jane in their own room, then Lake Park Home should perhaps consider providing a special room for this purpose, as is done in some long-term care facilities. (2)

While John and Mary Jane Brandt are a married couple, it is not hard to imagine a case in which two residents who are not married may wish to become sexually involved. Like the case of cohabitation, whether this kind of relationship is viewed as problematic will likely depend upon the sponsorship and values of the facility. If the administration of a facility feels obliged to exclude this kind of relationship among residents, it would do well to have a written policy in effect that is shared with prospective residents prior to admission.

CASE STUDY

Another case involving sexual activity at Lake Park Home is that of Mrs. Margaret Moore, aged 70. Margaret has a private room on the second floor of the facility. She is ambulatory but suffers from dementia due to Alzheimer's disease. Her husband, Glenn, faithfully comes to visit her every day in the afternoon. The nursing staff notices that Glenn sometimes closes the door to her room for about half an hour. When Glenn leaves, the staff always finds Margaret lying in bed although it is the middle of the afternoon. The staff strongly suspects that Glenn has been having sexual relations with his wife, and reports their suspicion to the facility's director of nursing. They wonder if his activity with his wife should be investigated further and perhaps stopped.

Sexual Activity Involving Residents with Dementia

The case of Margaret Moore again involves sexual relations between a husband and wife. However, there is a significant difference between this case and the former one. John and Mary Jane Brandt are both mentally competent, and presumably they are having sexual relations by mutual consent. Margaret Moore, on the other hand, is suffering from dementia.

It has been found that "residents with Alzheimer's disease and related disorders frequently maintain and express sexual feelings long into the disease process." (5) It has also been found that persons dealing with dementia in a spouse react in different ways to the continuation of a sexual relationship.

On the one hand, "some partners feel distressed about sexual overtures from a spouse who no longer knows their name or at times does not recognize who they are" and find troublesome "frequent sexual overtures (sometimes many each night) from partners who do not remember an episode of sexual intercourse that occurred earlier in the evening." (7) From another perspective, some male spouses may fear that a wife with dementia "is being forced into sex if she cannot consciously and verbally agree to sexual activity" and may be "troubled by feelings of guilt that they are taking advantage of or essentially raping their wives by continuing intercourse." (7) Moreover, some caregivers find the demands of caring for someone with a disease like Alzheimer's to "so deplete them physically and emotionally that they have little interest or energy for sex." (8) On the other hand, some spousal caregivers continue to find meaning and value in a sexual relationship as "one thing we can still do as a couple, one way we still feel close." (7)

From an ethical point of view, a major issue about a resident with dementia becoming involving in sexual activity is whether the resident can and does freely consent to participate in such activity. (4, 8, 9) In fact, a fundamental reason why rape is considered to be wrong is its non-consensual aspect. Such sexual activity involves invasion of bodily integrity and privacy.

It is important to keep in mind that dementia does not necessarily deprive an individual of all decision-making capabilities. For one thing, dementia may be episodic. The person suffering from dementia "will have good days and bad, lucid moments and confused." (10) Further, competency can be "context-specific." (4) Thus, it is not outside the realm of possibility that "the same patient who might be incapable of giving informed consent for medication or research, because of the complexity and novelty of information given, might be capable of giving informed consent to participate in a sexual relationship, a decision that is based more on old learning." (4)

It has also been suggested that a resident's present cognitive ability may not be the only relevant factor in judging the person's ability to enter into a sexual relationship. While persons suffering from dementia may be unable to recall past events, they may still be able to assign meaning to what they experience in the present and to reproduce meaningful relationships. Thus, the resident's ability to relate to other persons in the present is also a factor to consider. (8, 9)

The following sorts of questions may be helpful in evaluating the ability of a resident with dementia to choose to enter into a sexual relationship.

- Is the resident aware of who is initiating the sexual contact?

- Does the resident believe that the other person is a spouse and thus acquiesce out of a delusional belief, or is the resident cognizant of the other person's identity and intent?

- Can the patient state what level of sexual intimacy he or she would be comfortable with?

- Is the resident's behavior consistent with formerly held beliefs and values?

- Does the resident have the capacity to say no to any uninvited sexual contact? (4)

In sum, if a "resident exhibits behavior indicating lack of consent to the sexual activity, or if the attending physician or consulting psychiatrist/psychologist document that a resident is unable to consent," then it is ethically appropriate for staff to intervene to prevent this behavior. (5) On the other hand, staff must not prematurely assume that a resident is incapable of giving such consent just because he or she is suffering from dementia, but must carefully evaluate the resident and the situation.

CASE STUDY

Yet another troublesome case at the Lake Park Home involves the resident Gary Wagner, aged 78. Gary's wife died two years ago, before he entered the facility. It is obvious that Gary is still very much attracted to women. He makes a point of visiting with various women in the dining room, making flattering remarks. Of late Gary has been especially attracted to Thelma Murray. Thelma is somewhat confused but remains meticulous about her appearance and is always dressed very nicely. Thelma likes to spend time sitting in one of the facility's lounges in front of the fireplace, and Gary has started sitting next to her on the sofa with his arm around her. On one occasion when Thelma's daughter comes to visit her, she sees Gary repeatedly kissing her mother in the lounge. This upsets the daughter, who complains to the facility's administrator. After all, a nursing home is supposed to be a safe place for its residents!

Questions of Place

Although Thelma Murray is not suffering from a disease like Alzheimer's, she does exhibit some mental confusion. Thus, the issue of decisional capability for participating in sexual activity is again relevant. However, another facet of the case of Thelma and Gary is that the sexual activity is taking place in a public lounge area of the facility. Other residents may find such activity distracting and offensive, especially if they are using the lounge to visit with family or friends.

It has been pointed out that "proximity and intimacy in congregate settings may legitimately exclude some activities that could infringe either on the sensibilities of others or on the common good." (1) In an institutional setting, communal living space must be shared in a way that is respectful of all residents. Staff may cite this inevitable condition of living in a long-term care facility as justification for intervention in Gary Wagner's sexual advances towards female residents.

FOR GROUP DISCUSSION

1. In the case of Rita Tucker and Tim Shannon, it is left an open question whether Rita and Tim have a sexual relationship or whether their relationship is only one of companionship and mutual support. In your judgment, should the type of relationship they have enter into the decision whether they can live together in a long-term care facility?

   Suppose that Rita and Tim applied to a multi-level facility where they could share a two bedroom apartment in an assisted living unit. In your judgment, should this make a difference in whether they are allowed to share a living space in the facility?

2. Some long-term care facilities set aside a special room for married couples to carry on a sexual relationship. Should this room also be available to mentally competent but unmarried residents of the facility who request its use?

3. Suppose you are the director of nursing at the Lake Park Home. You find out that a pharmacy has just delivered to Leo Clark, a widower who lives in the residential unit, a prescription for a drug commonly used to enhance men's sex drives. Leo is able to take a trip outside the facility one day a week with one of his buddies from the neighborhood where he formerly lived. What, if anything, do you do about Leo having received the drug?

4. It has been suggested that a sexual history should be completed for each resident at the time of admission, especially those with dementia. (5, 8, 11) In terms of providing the optimal environment for residents, do you think it is useful to compile this kind of history? If so, what kinds of questions should be included? Are there questions that would be inappropriate to ask?

5. Construct hypothetical "what if" situations involving sexuality that could occur in a long-term care facility. For example, "What if a male resident reaches out and grabs your breast while you are trying to button his shirt?" Or, "What if a

resident mistakes another resident for his or her spouse and initiates intimate contact?" (In constructing your "what if" scenarios, you may wish to consult the description of range of sexual behaviors given at the beginning of this chapter.) Present and discuss your response for handling each hypothetical situation. As a group, you might also try to make a list of five or more appropriate responses to the situation and five or more inappropriate ways of responding. Finally, develop this "what if" exercise into one that can be used for staff training. (8, 11)

NOTES

1. American Association of Homes and Services for the Aging, "Sexual Activity in an AAHSA Facility," Timely Topics Series (Washington, DC: American Association of Homes and Services for the Aging).
2. Meredith Wallace, "Management of Sexual Relationships Among Elderly Residents of Long-term Care Facilities," *Geriatric Nursing* 13/6 (Nov./Dec. 1992): 308-11.
3. Susan Deacon, Victor Minichiello, David Plummer, "Sexuality and Older People: Revisiting the Assumptions," *Educational Gerontology* 21/5 (July/Aug. 1995): 497-513.
4. Peter A. Lichtenberg and Deborah M. Strzepek, "Assessments of Institutionalized Dementia Patients' Competencies to Participate in Intimate Relationships," *The Gerontologist* 30/1 (Feb. 1990): 117-20.
5. Philip Sloane, "Sexual Behavior in residents with dementia," *Contemporary Long Term Care* 16/10 (Oct. 1993): 66, 69, 108.
6. United States Catholic Conference, *Human Sexuality A Catholic Perspective for Education and Lifelong Learning* (Washington, DC: United States Catholic Conference, 1991).
7. Helen D. Davies, Antonette Zeiss, and Jared R. Tinklenberg, "'Till Death Do Us Part': Intimacy and Sexuality in The Marriages of Alzheimer's Patients," *Journal of Psychosocial Nursing* 30/11 (1992): 5-10.
8. Edna L. Ballard, "Sexuality in the Special Care Unit" in Stephanie B. Hoffman and Mary Kaplan (eds.), *Special Care Programs for People with Dementia* (Baltimore: Health Professions Press, 1996).
9. Athena M. McLean, "What Kind of Love Is This? When memory fades, desire lingers on. Can nursing homes cope with the residents' sexuality?" *The Sciences* (Sept./Oct. 1994): 36-39.
10. "Sexual Relations—'Mrs. Deere'" in Diane E. Hoffmann, Philip Boyle, and Steven A. Levenson, *Handbook for Nursing Home Ethics Committees* (Washington, DC: American Association of Homes and Services for the Aging, 1995).
11. Carly R. Hellen, "Intimacy: Nursing home resident issues and staff training," *The American Journal of Alzheimer's Disease* 10/2 (March/Arpil 1995): 12-17.

FOR FURTHER STUDY

- "Till Death Us Do Part: Married Life in Nursing Homes" and "A Single for Mr. Peterson to Die In" in Rosalie A. Kane and Arthur L. Caplan (eds.), *Everyday Ethics Resolving Dilemmas in Nursing Home Life* (New York: Springer, 1990).

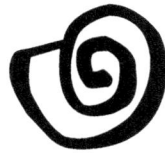

Chapter 7

Restraints

Restraints are "physical or chemical agents that are designed to inhibit voluntary movement" (1) on the part of residents. Governmental regulations define a "physical restraint" as "any manual method or physical or mechanical device, material, or equipment attached or adjacent to the resident's body that the individual cannot remove easily which restricts freedom of movement or normal access to one's body." (2) Examples of physical restraints are leg restraints, arm restraints, hand mitts, soft ties or vests, lap cushions, and lap trays that the resident cannot remove easily. Also included in the category of restraints are such practices as using side bed rails to keep a resident from voluntarily getting out of bed (as opposed to enhancing a resident's mobility while in bed), tucking in a sheet so tightly that a bed-bound resident's movement is restricted, using wheelchair safety bars to prevent a resident from rising out of the chair, placing a resident in a chair that prevents rising, or placing a chair or bed so close to a wall that the wall prevents the resident from rising out of the chair or voluntarily getting out of bed. (2, 3)

Governmental regulations define a "chemical restraint" as any drug that is used for discipline (that is, for the purpose of punishing or penalizing a resident) or for convenience (that is, to control a resident's behavior or manage it with a lesser amount of effort by the facility) and is not required to treat medical symptoms. (2) For example, a medication administered to quiet a resident who is disturbing other residents by crying out or by wandering qualifies as a restraint. (4)

At one time the use of restraints was a common and accepted practice in long-term care. Since the late 1980s, however, there has been a movement to change this practice. Some facilities have become "restraint free." Other facilities may still use restraints, but only occasionally and under carefully monitored conditions.

This chapter covers:
- *the original purposes for restraints;*
- *the harmful effects restraints have been found to have;*
- *current governmental regulations on the use of restraints;*
- *the ethical underpinning for reducing the use of restraints;*
- *who should make the decision about the use of restraints.*

CASE STUDY

Mrs. Marcella Cook, 83, has just been admitted to the Lancaster Community Care Center. Mrs. Cook is a widow, and her primary caregiver is her oldest son Doug, who lives in Lancaster.

Mrs. Cook is mentally alert but very frail, and has osteoporosis. When she is out of bed, she spends most of her time in a wheelchair. She is no longer steady on her feet, and prefers to lean on someone's arm when walking.

Like many facilities, the Lancaster Community Care Center does not have an over-abundance of staff. Although the staff is dedicated and conscientious, residents sometimes have to wait when they need help. Doug is very afraid that some day his mother will have to go to the bathroom and will try to get up and walk on her own because no staff member is available to help her. If this happens, Doug thinks there is a good chance that his mother will fall. Especially since she suffers from osteoporosis, a fall could easily result in broken bones for Mrs. Cook—bones that might be hard to heal at her age. Doug does not want his mother to be bedridden.

Doug asks the staff to put restraints on his mother while she is in the wheelchair to prevent her from getting out of the chair on her own and quite possibly falling. Kathy O'Brien, the director of nursing, meets with Doug and tells him that the facility does not like to use restraints unless absolutely necessary. Doug becomes angry, and accuses Kathy of not caring about the welfare of his mother. Doug makes it very clear that he thinks it is far more important for his mother to be protected from a fall than to undergo the indignity of having an accident and needing to be cleaned up. Further, Doug points out that state law requires him to wear a seat and shoulder belt while driving a car, and he doesn't see what the big fuss is about having "seat belts" on wheelchairs to protect elderly residents from harm. Doug ends his conversation with Kathy O'Brien by threatening to sue the facility for abuse and neglect if something is not done to restrain his mother.

In order to appease Doug, Kathy decides to place a wheelchair belt on Mrs. Cook on a trial basis. When this is done, Mrs. Cook becomes very agitated and starts crying.

Rethinking the Use of Restraints

In reviewing this case, our initial sympathies may lie with Mrs. Cook's son, Doug, rather than with the facility's director of nursing. After all, Doug's demand for restraints is an attempt to protect his mother from serious harm. We may well share Doug's puzzlement over the director of nursing's hesitancy to use a restraint on Mrs. Cook. As Doug points out, in some states individuals are required by law to use the restraint of a seat and shoulder belt when driving in order to be protected from harm, and this is a restriction that we as a society have accepted.

Originally, restraints were intended to serve three seemingly legitimate purposes. The first purpose was to protect the resident himself or herself from harm, such as injury from a fall. A second purpose was to enable medical procedures to be carried out for cognitively impaired residents who might, for example, pull out tubes. A third purpose was to protect other residents and staff from being harmed by a particular resident. (5, 6)

However, it has been found that the very use of restraints can have serious harmful consequences, both physically and psychologically, on the residents to whom they are applied. In a report on the use of restraints in long-term care facilities, the Council on Scientifc Affairs of the American Medical Association noted that

> Among the consequences of restraint application are physical risks, such as avoidable decline in the ability to ambulate, contractures, decreased muscle tone, increased risk of pressure sores and infections, constipation, and urinary incontinence or retention, and psychological risks, such as agitation, increase in disorganized behavior, depression, humiliation, fear of being abandoned, impaired self-image, and (in the presence of dementia) catastrophic reaction. (3)

Moreover, "other undesirable outcomes associated with restraint use are falls and injuries that ensue when individual residents attempt to personally remove restraints or try to climb over bed rails." (3) It has been estimated that "as many as 200 deaths occur annually as a result of strangulation or suffocation caused by restraints, even when they are correctly applied." (3) For example, residents have been "strangled after sliding down between a mattress and side rail while apparently trying to get out of bed." (7) In other cases residents have slid forward while sitting in a wheelchair or geriatric chair and been strangled by the restraining device. (7) Further, studies indicate that serious fall-related injuries are much more common in restrained residents than in those who are not restrained. (3)

The AMA's Council on Scientific Affairs has also noted the harmful effects of chemical restraints:

> Toxic reactions to these drugs, especially in the elderly, are well documented in the literature. Examples of these reactions are dizziness, tremors, tardive dyskinesia, increased agitation and confusion, dehydration, constipation, and urinary incontinence. In addition, studies showed that an increased risk for falls and hip fractures is associated with psychoactive drug use among the elderly. (3)

It is against this background that the Omnibus Budget Reconciliation Act of 1987 (OBRA) and the Health Care Financing Administration (HCFA) established regulations governing the use of restraints. These regulations (and subsequent clarifications of them) include the following standards for using restraints:

- The use of restraints is not totally excluded. However, restraint use must be limited to circumstances in which the resident has medical symptoms that warrant the use of restraints. In other words, the use of restraints must be a therapeutic intervention to attain and maintain the resident's highest practicable physical, mental, or psychosocial well-being.

- Residents have a right to be free from restraints imposed for the purpose of discipline (that is, for the purpose of punishing or penalizing a resident) or for the purpose of convenience (that is, to control a resident's behavior or manage a resident's behavior with a lesser amount of effort by the facility and not in the resident's best interest).

- The resident has a right to participate in the plan of care and to accept or refuse restraints. In order for the resident to make an informed decision, the facility must explain to the resident the potential risks and benefits of using a restraint, not using a restraint, and alternatives to restraint use.

- In the case of a resident who lacks decision-making capacity, the legal surrogate or other representative of the resident may make a decision about the use of restraints based on the same information that would have been provided to the resident.

- Medical symptoms that warrant the use of restraints must be documented in the resident's medical record, ongoing assessments, and care plans. There must be a physician's order reflecting the presence of a medical symptom.

- In the case of those residents whose care plans indicate the need for restraints, the facility must engage in a systematic and gradual process toward reducing restraints. (2, 3)

With the establishment of these regulations, long-term care facilities have looked for alternatives to the use of restraints and tried to create "restraint-free environments" for their residents. Indeed, the standards for long-term care developed by the Joint Commission on Accreditation of Healthcare Organizations now affirm that "the resident has a right to freedom from chemical or physical restraint" [RI.2.7] and that restraints should be "avoided if at all possible." [Intent of RI.2.7] (8) The following are examples of measures that may be taken to make restraint use unnecessary for a resident:

1. personal strengthening and rehabilitation program;

2. use of "personal assistance" devices such as hearing aids, visual aids and mobility device;

3. use of positioning devices such as body and seat cushions, and padded furniture;

4. efforts to design a safer physical environment, including the removal of obstacles that impede movement, placement of objects and furniture in familiar places, lower beds, and adequate lighting;

5. regular attention to toileting and other physical and personal needs, including thirst, hunger, the need for socialization, and the need for activities adapted to current abilities and past interests;

6. design of the physical environment to allow for close observation by staff;

7. efforts to increase staff awareness of residents' individual needs—possibly including assignment of staff to specific residents, in an effort to improve function and decrease difficult behaviors that might otherwise require the use of restraints;

8. design of resident living environments that are relaxing and comfortable, minimize noise, offer soothing music and appropriate lighting, and include massage, art or movement activities;

9. use of bed and chair alarms to alert staff when a resident needs assistance;

10. use of door alarms for residents who may wander away. (9)

How does this apply to the case of Mrs. Cook? Her son, Doug, may be anxious to have his mother restrained in her wheelchair because he is simply ignorant of the injuries which might come to his mother through the application of a physical restraint. Doug compares the restraint he wants placed on his mother to the use of a seat and shoulder belt in a car. However, the driver of a car controls the use of the belt and can remove it in an emergency situation. This is not true of the restraints applied to nursing home residents.

Considering the actions taken by the care center, it is clear that this situation was not well handled. First of all, there is no indication that any other methods were tried to prevent Mrs. Cook from trying to get up and walk on her own. For example, although the staff of the care center is very busy, they might make a point of inquiring about her toileting needs at certain intervals to prevent her from trying to get up to go to the bathroom on her own. Further, Mrs. Cook's physician was not consulted about restraining her. The director of nursing made the judgment to do this without the required written order from a physician indicating a genuine medical, therapeutic need for the restraint. Further, the restraint was applied at the request of Mrs. Cook's son, without Mrs. Cook herself being consulted. Since we have no indication that Mrs. Cook is suffering from a mental impairment that takes away her decision-making capability, the possible use of restraints should have been discussed with Mrs. Cook herself and her consent obtained to use them before the restraint was applied. We will return to the consent issue when discussing the ethics of using restraints.

Ethical Questions in the Use of Restraints

Thus far we have been working within the framework of governmental regulations. But what does ethics have to say about the use of restraints? From an ethical point of view, is it permissible to use restraints? If so, who appropriately makes the decision to use them? Is it ever ethically permissible to use restraints contrary to the wishes of the resident? And do the governmental regulations currently in place coincide with or differ from the ethical assessment of the use of restraints?

Is It Ethically Permissible to Use Restraints?

Health care providers have a duty of nonmaleficence to prevent harm from coming to patients and residents. At the same time, a principle of autonomy or self-determination is recognized; that is, the right of a patient or resident to make the final decision in matters pertaining to his or her own life and health care. The ethical question about using restraints has been posed in terms of a conflict between these two ethical principles:

> Since 1.6 million Americans currently reside in nursing homes, practices that govern the use of restraints in such facilities affect a sizable patient population. Moreover, the physical frailty and cognitive impairment of many of the residents of these facilities increase their vulnerability to bodily harm and create a conflict between the provision of a safe therapeutic environment and the right of the patient to basic liberty and self-determination. (5)

The main exceptions to a requirement of informed consent occur when the patient or others would be at risk for harm if the patient were not restrained. Under such circumstances, the resident's right of self-determination creates a conflict with the obligation of the long term care facility to provide a therapeutic environment that is safe for all residents of the facility. (5)

We have already seen that restraints can injure residents rather than protecting them from harm. This fact weakens the justification for placing restraints on grounds of nonmaleficence, at least as far as preventing harm to the resident himself or herself is concerned.

Exactly what are the implications of the ethical principle of autonomy for the use of restraints? It has been argued that the principle of autonomy creates a presumption against the use of restraints:

> The principle of autonomy holds that the elderly, even in the midst of frailty and dependency, should be free to determine the course and quality of their lives, to take risks, refuse treatment, control their daily lives as fully as possible. Thus, the principle of autonomy creates basic, nearly instinctive cautions against the use of physical and chemical restraints. For an ethic that challenges paternalistic bonds on patient *decision-making*, bonds on patient *mobility* are even more untenable. In autonomy-respecting care there would be a strong general presumption against the use of restraints. (10)

A presumption against the use of restraints finds further support in the negative impact restraint use has on the dignity of residents:

> In terms of dignity, physical restraints are problematic for a number of reasons. The public physical nature of these restraints is a powerful *social* statement. The presence of physical restraints can visibly identify residents as mentally incapacitated, physically untrustworthy, or behaviorally problematic. In the eyes of staff members, fellow residents, family members, even visitors who happen by, the physically restrained may be seen as publicly separated from the ranks of the responsible. Thus, in the secondary messages they give, restraints can produce a "pillory" effect, displaying the incapacities of the elderly in ways that give them sub-adult status.

> In terms of dignity, psychoactive drugs might seem preferable to physical restraints, but when used as chemical restraints these drugs can erode the basis of dignity—the individual's sense of self-possession and self-esteem. Residents can realize that they are being "medicated into" appropriate behavior, perhaps even into passivity and submission. Many staff members will know which residents are chemically restrained, and the tell-tale effects of such restraint may be clear to many others. In short, the dignity of the person can be seriously eroded by the restraining effects of psychoactive drugs. (10)

The eighteenth century philosopher Immanuel Kant formulated an ethical principle that "rational creatures should always treat other rational creatures as ends in themselves and never as only means to ends." (11) This principle is based on a belief that "every human being has an inherent worth resulting from the sheer possession of rationality." (11) Thus "we must always act in a way that respects this humanity in others and in ourselves." (11)   The loss of dignity suffered by residents who are restrained violates this ethical principle of respect for persons.

In sum, our ethical analysis supports the direction taken by current governmental regulations to reduce the use of restraints.

Who Decides about the Use of Restraints?

Suppose we are dealing with a situation where staff believes that the care of a particular resident cannot be satisfactorily addressed without the use of restraints. Can staff members themselves make the decision to ask a physician for an order to place restraints, even against the wishes of the resident and the family?

Ethically, the principle of autonomy is again relevant to answering this question. If a resident has the right to make the final decision in matters pertaining to his or her own life and health care, this entails that restraints should be used only with the consent of the resident. Further, it is recognized that the principle of autonomy allows an individual to refuse medical treatments. Since restraints are now considered a medical treatment modality, this entails that a mentally competent resident has the right to refuse the use of restraints and to assume any accompanying risks to his or her own personal safety. (5, 10)

Suppose, however, that the resident is mentally incapacitated. In such a case, consent for the placement of restraints should be sought from the resident's proxy decision maker rather than being made by staff alone. In making the decision, the proxy should be guided by the *principle of substituted judgment*. This principle directs the proxy to function as the resident's "other self," making a decision in accord with the resident's own values and wishes. In other words, the proxy should *not* do what he himself thinks is best for the resident, but should ask this question: Knowing the character of the resident, what would he or she say in this situation if mentally able to make a decision? Ethically, the principle of substituted judgment is the preferred standard for proxy decision making because it extends an individual's self-determination (that is, autonomy) into those situations in which the individual is no longer able to articulate his feelings.

Thus, the principle of autonomy provides an ethical grounding for the regulatory requirement that a "facility must obtain the resident's consent (or that of the legal representative) before physical restraints are used, unless the circumstances present an emergency." (10)

Could staff ever legitimately override the decision of a resident (or his proxy) to refuse the use of restraints? According to the libertarian principle proposed by the philosopher John Stuart Mill, an individual is free to take risks for himself; his liberty can be limited only to prevent him from harming other people. (12) Applying this principle to the case at hand, the placement of restraints against the wishes of the resident (or his proxy decision maker) might be ethically justified if the resident threatened serious harm to other residents or to staff and if there were no other means of dealing satisfactorily with the resident's behavior.

This kind of scenario is recognized in governmental regulations: "If a resident's unanticipated violent or aggressive behavior places him/her or others in imminent danger, the resident does not have the right to refuse the use of restraints." (2) Indeed, governmental regulations go beyond philosophical libertarianism to allow the application of restraints for the welfare of the resident himself. However, a caution is added: "In this situation, the use of restraints is a measure of last resort to protect the safety of the resident or others and must not extend beyond the immediate episode." (2)

In such circumstances, health care providers should try to find out what lies behind the resident's difficult behavior. (10) They should "search out the causes and subsurface messages of residents' harmful or disruptive behavior." (10) In particular, "restraints should not be a substitute for communication between the staff and the resident in question." (10) The goal of such communication should be "to understand the problematic behavior in question, then, where possible, to moderate and redirect it." (10) Again, restraints should not be misused as a quick fix in problem situations.

FOR GROUP DISCUSSION

1. Consider the following variations on the case of Mrs. Marcella Cook:

   A) Mrs. Cook is mentally alert but very frail and has osteoporosis. Recently, she broke her hip in a fall. It was surgically repaired at the hospital, and Mrs. Cook is now back at the Lancaster Community Care Center for the period of recuperation. What appropriate measures could and should be taken to try to protect Mrs. Cook from further falls? Should the use of restraints be considered in this case?

   B) Mrs. Cook is very frail, has osteoporosis, and now suffers from dementia. In addition, she recently broke her hip in a fall. It was surgically repaired at the hospital, and Mrs. Cook is back at the Lancaster Community Care Center for the period of recuperation. What appropriate measures could and should be taken to try to protect Mrs. Cook from further falls? Should the use of restraints be considered in this case?

2. In a white paper published by the American Association of Homes and Services for the Aging, it is suggested that a long-term care facility's policy on the use of restraints should " (a) identify the moral values and principles crucial to the facility's restraint policy; (b) indicate those uses which are contrary to the facility's philosophy of care; (c) discuss the alternatives to restraints which are favored by the facility; (d) delineate the conditions under which restraint use may be considered as a last resort; (e) spell out the decision-making, monitor-

ing, and documentation processes to be followed when restraints are in fact to be used." (4)

If you are connected with a long-term care facility, obtain a copy of the facility's policy on restraints and examine it according to the aforementioned criteria. Should any modifications be made of the policy? (If you are not connected with a long-term care facility, you might still obtain copies of the policies of several facilities and go through this exercise.)

NOTES

1. American Geriatrics Society, "Guidelines for Restraint Use" (revised January 1997), available at http://www.americangeriatrics.org/ .
2. *State Operations Manual* (Washington, DC: Department of Health and Human Services (DHHS) and Health Care Financing Administration (HCFA), 2000). Transmittal 20. Note that HCFA is now called Centers for Medicare and Medicaid Services (CMA).
3. Rosalie Guttman, Roy D. Altman, Mitchell S. Karlan, *Use of Restraints for Patients in Nursing Homes Report of the Council on Scientific Affairs of the American Medical Association, Archives of Family Medicine* 8 (1999): 101-5, available at http://archfami.ama-assn.org/
4. *Code Gray*, Case 2. Fanlight Productions (Boston, MA).
5. Council on Ethical and Judicial Affairs of the American Medical Association, "Guidelines for the Use of Restraints in Long Term Care Facilities" (June 1989) in *Reports* (Chicago: American Medical Association).
6. Rosalie A. Kane, "Ethical and Legal Issues in Long-Term Care: Food for Futuristic Thought," *Journal of Long-Term Care Administration* (Fall 1993): 66-74.
7. U.S. Food and Drug Administration, "Safe Use of Physical Restraint Devices," a FDA Backgrounder available at http://www.fda.gov/ .
8. Joint Commission on Accreditation of Healthcare Organizations, 2002-2003 *Standards for Long Term Care* (Oakbrook Terrace, IL: Joint Commission Resources, 2002).
9. Minnesota Department of Health, "Safety Without Restraints" http://www.health.state.mn.us/divs/fpc/safety.htm
10. Bart J. Collophy, "The Use of Restraints in Long-Term Care: The Ethical Issues" (Washington, DC: American Association of Homes and Services for the Aging, 1992).
11. William H. Shaw, "Normative Theories of Ethics" in William H. Shaw (ed.), *Social and Personal Ethics*, 2nd ed. (Belmont, CA: Wadsworth, 1996).
12. John Stuart Mill, "On Liberty" in *The Utilitarians* (Garden City, NY: Anchor/Doubleday, 1973).

FOR FURTHER STUDY

- "Restraints—'Mrs. Quick'" in Diane E. Hoffmann, Philip Boyle, and Steven A. Levenson, *Handbook for Nursing Home Ethics Committees* (Washington, DC: American Association of Homes and Services for the Aging, 1995).

- "Let My Persons Go! Restraints of the Trade" in Rosalie A. Kane and Arthur L. Caplan (eds.), *Everyday Ethics Resolving Dilemmas in Nursing Home Life* (New York: Springer, 1990).

- Judith V. Braun and Steven Lispon (eds.), *Toward a Restraint-Free Environment: Reducing the Use of Physical and Chemical Restraints in Long-Term and Acute Care Settings* (Baltimore, MD: Health Professions Press, 1993).

Part Two

Ethical Issues at the End of Life

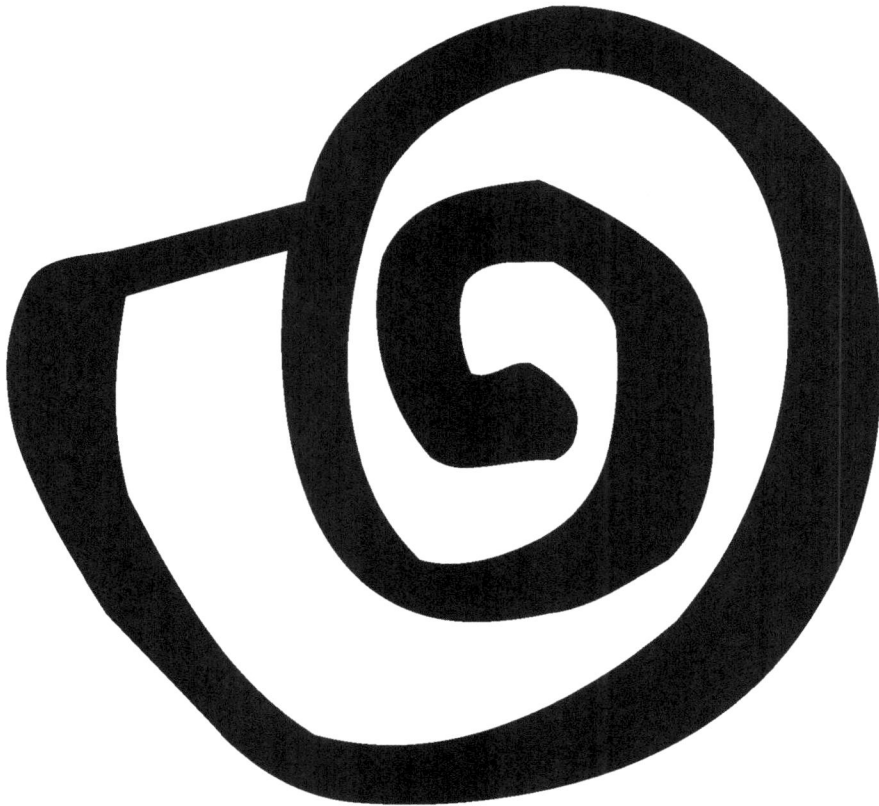

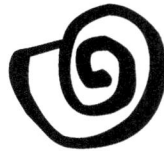

Chapter 8

Making Decisions about Using or Forgoing Life-Sustaining Treatments

A life-sustaining treatment is "any medical intervention, technology, procedure, or medication that is administered to a patient in order to forestall the moment of death, whether or not the treatment is intended to affect the underlying life-threatening disease(s) or biologic processes." (1) Examples include chemotherapy, kidney dialysis, resuscitation, the use of a ventilator, and tube feeding. The administration of antibiotics or blood pressure medication can also fall into this category in some cases.

This chapter covers:
- *how to make decisions about using or forgoing life-sustaining treatments;*
- *whether it is permissible to withdraw a treatment once it has been started;*
- *the difference between forgoing a life-sustaining treatment and euthanasia;*
- *who should make decisions on behalf of incapacitated residents;*
- *how proxy decision makers should come to a treatment decision.*

CASE STUDY

Ray and Lynn Fulton, both 76, have been residents of the St. Francis Home, a multi-level care facility, for a year. Three years ago Ray had a cancerous tumor in his stomach, but chemotherapy had worked in shrinking it and causing the cancer to go into remission. However, within the last month the cancer has recurred.

Chemotherapy is promptly begun for Ray. However, Ray's doctor is honest with him that, this time around, the chemotherapy will probably slow the growth of the tumor and prolong his life but is not likely to "cure" his cancer as it did before.

The first time Ray had cancer, he had tolerated the chemotherapy treatments reasonably well. But this time he experiences nausea and vomiting, and feels so "washed out" for a week after each treatment that he cannot even enjoy his grandchildren when they come to visit him. In addition, the pain from the cancer is considerable.

To make things worse, two months later Ray develops pneumonia. Because of his overall weakened physical condition, Ray's physician recommends hospitalization with antibiotic treatment and placement on a ventilator for assistance in breathing. Ray, however, tells his doctor and his wife that he doesn't want any of this. In fact, Ray tells them that he wants to stop chemotherapy treatments as well. These treatments are, he says, only prolonging his suffering. He states that he has lived a full life, and is ready to die. Ray had been a very successful attorney, and no one doubts that he is still sharp mentally.

Ray and Lynn have three children. Two of the children support Ray's decision to forgo all medical treatments, but his wife Lynn and one of their daughters disagree and feel that Ray has "given up too soon." After all, he beat the odds with cancer once before, and he has grandchildren to live for and enjoy.

Lynn asks the chaplain at the St. Francis Home, Father Morris, to visit Ray and talk with him about his situation. Lynn knows that Ray respects the chaplain and will listen to him. However, when Father Morris learns more details about Ray's case, he himself wonders what is the right thing to do. He is not sure that he should try to persuade Ray to continue with life-sustaining treatments. Perhaps his role is to help Ray prepare for death.

Ethical Principles for Making Decisions about Life-Sustaining Treatments

Two ethical principles are commonly brought into discussions about using or forgoing life-sustaining treatments: the *principle of patient autonomy* and the *principle of weighing benefits and burdens*.

At one time the practice of medicine was considered "paternalistic." The physician made the treatment decisions and the patient and family members went along with the decision without question. This model of medical practice has changed. Now there is a commitment to *patient autonomy*; to patient self-determination. Patient autonomy entails that a patient has a right to be involved in decision making about medical treatments, and indeed, to make the final decision about using or forgoing treatments.

In the case of Ray Fulton, there is no doubt that he is "competent"; that is, he is mentally capable of making treatment decisions. Ray has clearly expressed his desire to forgo treatments for his pneumonia and to have the chemotherapy stopped. According to the principle of patient autonomy, Ray's physician should agree to his wishes and not give these treatments.

Sometimes the principle of patient autonomy is presented in such a way that health care providers are expected to abide by the wishes of the patient no matter what he wants and no matter what the rationale for his decision. This is probably an extreme reaction to the paternalism once practiced in medicine. Experience with putting the principle of patient autonomy into practice is causing us to recognize certain limitations to patient choices. One of these limitations is the expectation that patients should make their treatment decisions in accord with the accepted principles of health care ethics.

Historically, a distinction was made between ordinary and extraordinary medical treatments. The accompanying moral principle stated that ordinary treatments must always be provided when needed but that we do not have an obligation to use treatments which are extraordinary. Aspirin, blood pressure medication, and antibiotics might be considered ordinary treatments. Ventilators, chemotherapy, and kidney dialysis might be given as examples of extraordinary treatments.

However, ethicists came to see problems with this distinction and the accompanying moral principle. Recently, ethicists have refined it into a *principle of weighing benefits and burdens*. This is not a completely new standard. Rather, it is an attempt to introduce clarity and precision into our discussions by focusing on one of the traditional interpretations of the ordinary/extraordinary treatment distinction. (2)

According to the principle of weighing benefits and burdens, there are two cases in which it is morally permissible to forgo (that is, to withhold or withdraw) a life-sustaining treatment:

- when the burdens of the treatment outweigh its benefits;
- when the treatment is useless or futile, providing no benefit to the patient.

The first part of this principle is something like a cost/benefit analysis. What are the benefits the treatment might bring? Will it bring about a cure (or even a partial cure) for the patient? Will it give the patient relief from pain? Will it increase the patient's physical mobility? Will it restore the patient's consciousness? Will it enhance the patient's ability to communicate with family and friends? On the other hand, are some aspects of the proposed treatment burdensome? Will the treatment itself cause the patient pain or substantial discomfort? Will the treatment entail any psychological burdens, such as depression? Will the patient have difficulty getting access to the treatment? (For example, will the patient have to drive a substantial distance each week to get the treatment?) Will the patient have to be restrained to tolerate the treatment? (For example, will the patient have to be restrained to prevent him from pulling out a feeding tube?) Will the treatment impose a financial burden on the patient or his family?

Balancing the sides, are the benefits of the treatment greater than the burdens? If the answer is yes, then the treatment should be undertaken. On the other hand, are the burdens greater than the benefits? Then it is morally permissible to forgo the treatment.

It should be noted that our interpretation of the principle of weighing benefits and burdens includes benefits and burdens both for the patient (e.g., increasing the patient's physical mobility) and for other people (e.g., the cost of the treatment for the patient's family). It also includes benefits and burdens of both a purely medical nature (e.g., pain and discomfort caused by the treatment) and a non-medical nature (e.g., the cost of treatment). What is more controversial is the inclusion of quality of life considerations. Should we consider the burdensomeness *of the life sustained* through a treatment or should we limit ourselves to consideration of the burdensomeness *of the treatment itself*? (2) Consider, for example, the case of Ray Fulton. The administration of antibiotics for his pneumonia may not in itself be particularly burdensome. However, treating his pneumonia will prolong his battle with cancer and the suffering of his dying process. In other words, the administration of antibiotics will prolong a life which has itself become burdensome. Indeed, pneumonia was at one time called "the old person's friend" because it brought about death for persons suffering from other debilitating diseases.

In some cases a treatment simply will not work physically for a patient. For example, some patients cannot tolerate tube feeding because of a heart condition. Or again, antibiotics are ineffective against some types of pneumonia. In such cases, the treatment provides no benefit whatever to the patient. The second part of the principle of weighing benefits and burdens states that when a treatment is useless or futile, there is no moral obligation to use it. Suppose, for example, that chemotherapy would prove ineffective in stopping the growth of Ray's cancerous tumor. In that event, there would be no obligation to continue the treatment.

When using the principle of weighing benefits and burdens to make decisions about life-sustaining treatments, decisions are made on a case-by-case basis. There is no treatment which must automatically be used. Likewise, there is no treatment which can automatically be forgone. The question to ask is: What will this treatment do for this particular patient who is in this particular condition? Even if a treatment is commonly available (such as antibiotics), there is not necessarily a moral obligation to use it.

In discussing life-sustaining treatments, we have spoken of both the principle of patient autonomy and the principle of weighing benefits and burdens. Is there a way of putting them together? While it is true that we should abide by the wishes of the patient, it is also true that patients should not make their decisions in a purely arbitrary way. We should encourage them and help them to look at the relative benefits and burdens of the treatment, and to make their decision on that basis.

How does all of this apply to the case of Ray Fulton? We have already discussed the use of antibiotics for his pneumonia, but what about his desire to stop chemotherapy treatments? Do the benefits and burdens of the chemotherapy justify stopping this treatment? The chemotherapy is not expected to cure Ray's cancer. It is expected to slow the growth of the tumor and hence to prolong Ray's life, although we do not know for how long a time. Thus, while there is some benefit to Ray from the chemotherapy, the benefit is limited. On the other hand, the chemotherapy has some definitely burdensome aspects to it. Ray is experiencing nausea and vomiting from the chemotherapy, and treatments leave him feeling so "washed out" for a whole week that he cannot even enjoy his grandchildren when they come to visit him. Further, it is said that the pain Ray is experiencing from the cancer is considerable, and prolonging his life through administration of chemotherapy is only prolonging this pain. In addition, there are the costs of continued aggressive treatment to consider, not only the chemotherapy treatments themselves but the fact that Ray must be placed in a unit of St. Francis Home which provides a higher level of nursing care and hence is more expensive. Ray may worry about what will happen to his wife Lynn if their financial resources are depleted. In sum, in this case it would be reasonable to judge that the burdens of Ray's chemotherapy treatments outweigh the benefits, and thus stopping the chemotherapy treatments is a morally permissible course of action.

Common Misconceptions about Forgoing Life-Sustaining Treatments

The case of Ray Fulton involves not starting treatments for his pneumonia and stopping chemotherapy for his cancer. In the past, some have made a distinction between *withholding* a life-sustaining treatment (that is, never starting a treatment) and *withdrawing* a treatment (that is, stopping a treatment). Some judged that it is morally permissible to withhold a treatment but that, once started, a treatment cannot be stopped. This kind of thinking has changed. Ethically, it is now considered just as permissible to withdraw a treatment as never to start it.

Why has this change in attitude taken place? In some cases we may not be sure, in advance of using a life-sustaining treatment, whether it will benefit the patient or not. If we have the mentality "once a treatment is started, it cannot be stopped," we may be afraid to try the treatment. This is because we would not want to be locked into a treatment which will not help the patient but will only prolong his dying process and suffering. Suppose we adopt a policy across the board of forgoing a treatment when its benefits are uncertain. This might mean that there are patients who would have benefited from the treatment who will never receive it and whose lives will be lost. Thus, time-limited trials of life-sustaining treatments are recommended. If it is unclear whether a treatment will benefit a patient, it should be tried out for a predetermined period of time and its effect evaluated. If it proves not to work physically or to be more burdensome than beneficial to the patient, then we should feel free to withdraw it. (1)

It may be more difficult psychologically for family members or health care workers to stop a treatment than never to start it. But if we have tried a treatment and then decide to withdraw it for lack of beneficial results, we can at least feel that we have done everything we can to help the patient.

Some family members or health care workers may feel guilty about withdrawing a life-sustaining treatment. The reason is that they feel they will be doing something to cause the death of the patient. In other words, they are afraid that, in stopping a life-sustaining treatment, they will be engaging in an act of euthanasia. This fear is unfounded. It is important to keep in mind that there is some underlying disease—more technically speaking, an underlying fatal pathology—which made the use of the life-sustaining treatment necessary in the first place. And it is this underlying disease that will cause the patient's death when the life-sustaining treatment is removed. In the case of Ray Fulton, it is the stomach cancer that made it necessary to start chemotherapy. And it is the cancer that will cause his death when he is taken off the chemotherapy.

Another common misconception about decisions to forgo life-sustaining treatment is that, once such a decision has been made, health care providers will abandon the patient. This is not true. Pain medication and comfort care will still be provided. A slogan has recently surfaced in health care, "Care, not cure." A time will come in a patient's illness when nothing more can be done medically to help the patient recover from the disease. At this stage the emphasis changes to one of relieving the symptoms of the disease and of enabling the patient to spend his final days in as comfortable and meaningful a way as possible.

Finally, if a decision has been made to stop treatment, this does not mean that the treatment must be withdrawn immediately thereafter. Time can be provided for family members and friends to say final good-byes and for religious rituals to take place before the treatment is stopped and the patient is allowed to die.

Decisions in the Case of Mentally Incapacitated Patients

Ray Fulton is still able to make his own health care decisions. But suppose that, in addition to cancer and pneumonia, Ray was also suffering from severe dementia. Who should make the decisions about continuing or discontinuing chemotherapy and about providing or refusing the doctor's recommended treatments for pneumonia? And on what basis should these decisions be made?

A *surrogate* or *proxy decision maker* is someone who makes health care decisions for a patient who is not mentally competent to do so. The patient's next of kin often fulfills this role, but another relative, a close friend, or an individual who knows the patient well may serve in this capacity. Often one of these individuals naturally emerges as the proxy decision maker. For example, in the case of Ray Fulton it would be natural for his wife to be called upon to make treatment decisions on his behalf. However, it is now possible for a patient to go beyond informal arrangements and to select in advance an individual who will be legally recognized as his proxy decision maker. This is done by executing the legal document known as a *durable power of attorney for health care* (see the chapter on "Advance Directives"). If a patient has not been able to execute this document, it is possible for a court to appoint a guardian to serve legally as the patient's proxy decision maker. When a patient is mentally incapable of making his own treatment decisions and a proxy decision maker must be found, the first step health care providers should take is to determine if the patient has executed a durable power of attorney for health care or has a legally appointed guardian. This information should be noted in the patient's medical records.

How should a proxy decision maker go about making his decision on behalf of the patient? The preferred standard for proxy decision making is the *principle of substituted judgment*. In this case, the proxy decision maker knows the patient well enough to be able to predict what the patient would want in the case at hand if the patient were able to make a judgment. In other words, the proxy decision maker makes a decision in accord with the values and desires of the patient. The proxy should ask: How would the patient judge the respective benefits and burdens of the treatment? The answer to this question should serve as the basis for making the decision to use or forgo the treatment. Stipulations in advance directives, conversations with the patient, and knowledge of the patient's behavior and choices throughout his life can all serve as indicators of what the patient himself would want done.

Let's suppose that Lynn Fulton were serving as the proxy decision maker on behalf of her husband Ray. As the case is described above, she wants Ray's life saved and treatments for his pneumonia and cancer provided. However, as his proxy decision maker Lynn should be thinking in terms of what Ray himself would want.

There are some cases in which the standard of substituted judgment cannot be applied. This is so if the patient has never been mentally competent during his lifetime and thus was never able to express any preferences. This is also true if the patient no longer has any close living relatives or friends who know him well. In such cases the *best interests standard* must be used. According to this standard, the proxy attempts to assess objectively what is the best option for the patient. Weighing benefits and burdens of a treatment can be used as a guideline in making this assessment.

It is important to keep in mind, however, that the principle of substituted judgment is the preferred standard whenever it can be used. Making proxy decisions in accord with the wishes and values of the patient is an extension of the principle of patient autonomy.

FOR GROUP DISCUSSION

1. Have you ever experienced in your own family or with close friends a situation in which a decision had to be made about using or forgoing life-sustaining treatments? Describe the case and the decision that was made. Why was this particular decision made? If the decision had been up to you, would you have made the same decision or a different one? Why or why not? Did any of the ethical principles presented in this chapter figure into the decision-making process, at least implicitly?

2. One of the functions of an ethics committee can be *retrospective review* of the decisions that have in fact been made about using or forgoing life-sustaining treatments within a facility over a period of time. This is done as a matter of quality control and to determine if any patterns emerge indicating problems that need to be addressed.

   Suppose that you are a member of the ethics committee of the Cedarville Care Facility and that the following cases are brought to the committee for retrospective review. In each case, is the decision that has been made consistent with the ethical principles governing the use and forgoing of life-sustaining treatments? (Note that, when such reviews are conducted, the names of residents may be suppressed in the presentation of the cases to the ethics committee in order to respect resident confidentiality.)

   • A female resident, 78, had moderate dementia. She began to suffer kidney failure, and a decision had to be made about putting her on dialysis. The resident's daughter was her legally designated proxy decision maker. The daughter decided against dialysis being undertaken. Her daughter stated that her mother had always been an avid reader, and believed that her mother would not want to be kept alive when she no longer "has her mind."

   • A male resident, 76, needed blood transfusions about twice a month. His prognosis was good if he had them. However, he was a very independent individual, and made it clear to the nursing staff that he would "rather die than have needles stuck in him all the time." The staff decided not to try to pressure him into agreeing to the transfusions.

- A female resident, 40 years old, was suffering from some paralysis and had much reduced mental capacity due to serious brain damage in an automobile accident. She had never married, and her parents, themselves in their early seventies, were her legal guardians. Prior to the accident, she had been a high school science teacher. She had done a lot of reading, had organized a science club for her students, and had arranged numerous field trips. Her students and her teaching were "her whole life."

  At one point her blood pressure became dangerously low. Given her overall condition, her physician discussed with her parents whether medication should be administered to keep up her blood pressure. Without hesitation, her parents affirmed that the medication should be given to her. They stated that, as parents, they just couldn't "bury their own daughter."

3. The case of Ray Fulton represents a conflict situation pertaining to the use of life-sustaining treatments. Ray, the patient in question, wishes to forgo all further medical treatments, and two of his children support his position. On the other hand, Ray's wife Lynn and one of their daughters disagree with Ray's decision.

   In American medical ethics, emphasis is placed on individual autonomy. Following this principle, it would be concluded that health care providers should do what Ray wants, even if family members cannot accept his decision. Some contend, however, that an exclusive emphasis on individual autonomy represents an extreme form of individualism that ignores the fact that we are involved in relationships with other people and that our actions as individuals also affect them.

   In your view, should Ray's wife and children have any say in the decision about using or forgoing further medical treatments? If so, what do you think their appropriate role is? Do you think that the ethical principle of autonomy should be refined in any way? (In discussing these questions you may find it helpful to read the description of the *ethics of care* in the Appendix.)

4. If an individual is not mentally capable of making medical treatment decisions, then it is standard practice to resort to a proxy decision maker. However, it may be difficult in practice to determine when a proxy decision maker is needed. For example, in a long-term care facility one is likely to be dealing with residents suffering from dementia in varying degrees. These persons may be able to make some kinds of decisions but not others. What indications would you look for to determine if a resident is still capable of making important life-and-death decisions about using or forgoing medical treatments?

NOTES

1. Hastings Center, *Guidelines on the Termination of Life-Sustaining Treatment and the Care of the Dying* (Briarcliff Manor, NY: Hastings Center, 1987).
2. President's Commission for the Study of Ethical Problems in Medicine and Biomedical and Behavioral Research, *Deciding to Forego Life-Sustaining Treatment* (1983; reprint New York: Concern for Dying).

3. Orville N. Griese, *Catholic Identity in Health Care: Principles and Practice* (Braintree, MA: Pope John Center, 1987).

FOR FURTHER STUDY

*   President's Commission for the Study of Ethical Problems in Medicine and Biomedical and Behavioral Research, *Deciding to Forego Life-Sustaining Treatment* March 1983 (reprint New York: Concern for Dying), pp. 73-77, 82-89.

*   Hastings Center, *Guidelines on the Termination of Life-Sustaining Treatment and the Care of the Dying* (Briarcliff Manor, NY: Hastings Center, 1987), Introduction and Part One.

*   Joanne Lynn and Joan Harrold, *Handbook for Mortals* (New York: Oxford, 1999). This book provides a comprehensive guide to end of life care written for a general audience. It offers a wealth of practical advice on such issues as how to make decisions about care, where to find support and treatment resources, how to communicate with physicians, withdrawing life-sustaining treatment, how to get effective pain management, and palliative nutrition. Both co-authors are themselves physicians. Dr. Lynn is director of the Center to Improve Care of the Dying at George Washington University.

*   Joseph Cardinal Bernardin, *The Gift of Peace* (Chicago: Loyola Press, 1997). This is an autobiographical account of the experience of dying from cancer written from a religious perspective. It includes a description of Bernardin's eventual decision to forgo further life-sustaining treatments.

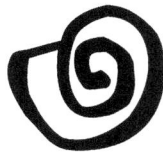

Chapter 9

Resuscitation

Cardiopulmonary resuscitation (CPR) as practiced in a health care facility is a much more extensive and invasive procedure than the resuscitation taught to members of the community by the Red Cross. It may include such procedures as chest compression, administration of various medications, electrical shocks to restart the heart, placement of a breathing tube (intubation), and placement on a breathing machine (ventilator). Patients may suffer serious bruises or broken ribs during resuscitation attempts.

Initially, CPR was used on otherwise healthy individuals who experienced cardiac or respiratory arrest during surgery or as a result of near-drowning. Today CPR is routinely administered in health care settings to patients who experience cardiopulmonary arrest. Since cessation of heart beat and respiration is a normal part of the dying process, CPR can potentially be used on every individual prior to death. In fact, the frequent performance of CPR on patients who are terminally ill or who have little chance of surviving for more than a brief period of time has caused concern that CPR is being used too extensively. (1) This, in turn, has led to *DNR (do not resuscitate) orders,* alternately called *DNAR (do not attempt resuscitation) orders* or *no CPR orders.* (2)

Some people do not realize that attempts at resuscitation do not always work. The Council on Ethical and Judicial Affairs of the American Medical Association reports that, of the patients who receive CPR, only one third survive the resuscitation effort, and only one third of these individuals, in turn, survive until discharge from the hospital. (1) Studies show that a significant number of people change their minds about wanting CPR when they learn the actual success rates of this procedure. (3, 4)

This chapter covers:
- *applying the ethical principle of patient autonomy to resuscitation decisions;*
- *applying the principle of weighing benefits and burdens to resuscitation decisions;*
- *DNR orders in long-term care facilities;*
- *DNR orders during surgery;*
- *DNR orders when resuscitation would be futile;*
- *the relation of DNR orders to advance directives;*
- *EMS personnel honoring DNR orders.*

Ethical Principles for Using or Forgoing Resuscitation

Decisions about attempting or withholding resuscitation are decisions about using or forgoing a life-sustaining treatment. Thus, such decisions involve applying principles presented in the chapter "Making Decisions about Using or Forgoing Life-Sustaining Treatments"; namely, the principle of autonomy and the principle of weighing benefits and burdens.

At one time, physicians usually made the decision about using or forgoing resuscitation. However, it is now standard practice that the patient (or the appropriate proxy decision maker) make the final decision after discussion with the physician. This change in practice reflects the current emphasis on patient autonomy. The patient (or proxy) should be guided in this decision by the principle of weighing benefits and burdens; namely, that it is morally permissible to forgo resuscitation if resuscitation (and its results) would prove futile or more burdensome than beneficial.

The following case studies will illustrate particular dilemmas about resuscitation that have been troubling to health care providers. The two aforementioned ethical principles will be applied to these dilemmas.

CASE STUDY

Martha Thompson, 78, is mentally alert but confined to a wheel chair since one of her legs was amputated a year ago. In spite of the efforts of an occupational therapist to adapt her home to her new needs, Martha is not coping well. Her children are considering placing her in a nursing home. When Martha's children inquire about admission to Sunset Park Care Facility, the administrator tells them that all residents of the facility agree to forgo resuscitation in the event of cardiopulmonary arrest. Since Martha is still quite alert mentally and able to enjoy many activities, her family is not sure that having a DNR order for her would be the right thing to do. At the same time, Sunset Park is the closest long-term care facility, and having Martha there would allow her children to visit her frequently. Martha's children wonder about the fairness of the facility's blanket policy on resuscitation.

Resuscitation in Long-Term Care

The case of Martha involves a requirement that all residents of a long-term care facility have a DNR order. By federal regulation, this can no longer be done. According to the Centers for Medicare and Medicaid Services (formerly HCFA), "Any Medicaid or Medicare certified and/or participating provider which operates under a policy or procedure which denies resuscitation to all patients is in violation of the Medicare residents rights and/or quality of care requirements." (5) In fact, while nursing homes used to call 911 for Emergency Medical Technicians (EMTs) to come to administer CPR, the new regulations mandate that long-term care facilities have staff trained to administer CPR on-site. (5) The thinking underlying these regulations is that each person has a right to choose to have or to forgo resuscitation. From an ethical point of view, these regulations place a premium on patient autonomy.

Long-term care facilities serve primarily the older adult population. To take the position that anyone over a certain age should automatically be denied CPR could be considered discriminatory and an instance of ageism. It would be like saying that anyone who is physically or mentally disabled should automatically be denied resuscitation. In both cases, what is relevant is whether the individual has some underlying disease which, in whomever it might be found, makes a decision not to resuscitate a reasonable one. If the underlying disease would make resuscitation (and its effects) more burdensome than beneficial, or would make resuscitation attempts futile, then and only then is it morally permissible for a DNR order to be written.

CASE STUDY

Art Melloy, 94, has been a resident of the Monmouth Care Center for ten years. In spite of his age, he is in fairly good health. Although he sometimes "lives in the past," he is generally alert mentally.

Art keeps joking with the care center's staff that they should start preparing for a big 100th birthday celebration for him. Indeed, his own father, who was a farmer, had lived to the ripe old age of 102!

Several years ago a DNR order was written for Art. Although he still enjoys life, he consented to the DNR order because he believes that, if his heart should naturally stop or if he should stop breathing, this is God's way of saying that it is time for him "to go home to heaven."

Because Art has developed some heart problems, his physician recommends implantation of a pacemaker. Art agrees to have this procedure performed. However, his youngest daughter, who is a nurse by profession, wonders about the status of her father's DNR order. She knows that doctors do not like to let people die during surgery. She wonders if an attempt will be made to resuscitate her father at the hospital if, by chance, he should suffer an arrest during surgery.

Resuscitation in the Operating Room

Another issue that has arisen is the status of DNR orders in the operating room, DNR in the OR. During surgery, "the patient is subject to anesthesia and trauma, which can cause cardiopulmonary arrest even in an individual who might be at relatively low risk outside the OR." (6) Since the cause of arrest in these circumstances is not an underlying disease but factors introduced by the surgical procedure, some have thought that a DNR order should be suspended in the operating room. Indeed, if a patient does not want to survive the surgical procedure, what is the point of undergoing it?

Recently, however, "the practice of suspending DNR orders in the OR has been challenged on ethical grounds." (6) Calling on the principle of weighing benefits and burdens, some have pointed out that "the risks and benefits of resuscitation must be weighed as they are in any setting..." (6) On the one hand, "a patient undergoing curative or therapeutic surgery, such as coronary artery bypass grafting," would likely want resuscitation since "he could look forward to improved survival and quality of life once he made it through the operation." (6) On the other hand, "a patient whose planned surgery is palliative—for example, a patient with end-stage cancer undergoing a colon resection to relieve pain and vomiting caused by severe obstruction—may prefer that the OR team not intervene if he arrests." (6)

Consider the case of Art, a 94-year-old man undergoing the surgical implantation of a pacemaker for his heart. A person of this age who survives resuscitation "is likely to require an ICU stay and life support measures." (6) And with the resuscitation attempt, there is the possibility that he might be left with serious brain injury. Hence, if this patient survives resuscitation, he might be in a much worse condition than before the arrest. (6) Weighing the possible benefits and burdens of resuscitation for Art, it may be a reasonable decision that the DNR order should remain in effect during surgery.

Furthermore, it has been argued that automatically suspending DNR orders during procedures involving anesthesia "may not sufficiently address a patient's rights to self-determination in a responsible and ethical manner." (7) The phraseology "patient self-determination" is another way of expressing the concept of patient autonomy. A "patient doesn't lose his right to refuse treatment when he enters the OR." (6) Thus, physicians are now increasingly consulting with patients (or their proxy decision makers) prior to surgery about maintaining or suspending a DNR order during surgery and the period of recovery immediately thereafter.

CASE STUDY

Roger Murray, 67, has been battling colon cancer for three years. Throughout this time he has tried to stay active and live as normal a life as possible. He has remained as manager of the sporting goods store he started many years ago, has played golf several times a week, and has continued to teach religious education classes to children in his church.

However, chemotherapy is no longer keeping the cancer in check. It has now spread to other organs in Roger's gastrointestinal system. In several months, Roger experiences a weight loss of fifty pounds. He feels so "wiped out" all the time that he finally has to retire from his business and give up most of his other regular activities. He spends most of the time at home. And the pain from his cancer is becoming considerable.

Roger can tell that the responsibilities of caring for him are putting a strain on his wife. For this reason he decides to go to the Hudson Care Facility. Upon entering the nursing home, Roger is given a thorough exam by his doctor, who tells him that he has begun the "final downhill slide." His physician advises him to have a DNR order written. A cardiopulmonary arrest, his doctor says, would simply be a part of his body giving out in the dying process. CPR might not work at all in restoring Roger's heart beat and respiration, and even if it did, Roger would likely suffer another arrest in a few days.

Roger, however, refuses to consent to a DNR order. He believes that God can work miracles for those who believe in him. In Roger's view, deciding to forgo resuscitation—just standing by and allowing death to come—would show a lack of faith in God's power to heal. Roger repeatedly tells the staff at the Hudson Care Facility—including the administrator, the director of nursing, and the person in charge of the facility's medical records—that he wants all available treatments, including resuscitation. Roger's wife and children support him wholeheartedly in this decision.

Roger's physician feels strongly that additional therapy, including CPR, would be futile and a waste of medical resources, and should not be provided. He decides to write a DNR order on Roger's chart. This is a case, he believes, in which "the doctor knows best" and the patient and family are acting irrationally.

However, when a resident advocate at the care facility learns what has happened, she feels very uncomfortable about a DNR order having been written contrary to the wishes of the resident. She decides to go over the doctor's head and take the case to the facility's ethics committee.

Resuscitation and Judgments of Futility

In the case of Roger, a physician unilaterally writes a DNR order, against the expressed wishes of the patient, because he believes attempting resuscitation would be futile. According to the *principle of weighing benefits and burdens*, it is morally permissible to forgo a life-sustaining treatment if it would be *futile or useless in nature*, essentially providing no benefit to the patient. On the other hand, unilateral DNR orders on the part of physicians represent a serious restriction on patient autonomy.

Such a practice might be defended on the grounds that patient self-determination is meaningful only when the patient is presented with a choice between medically viable options, and a futile treatment is not really a viable option. (8, 9, 10) Further, this practice might be defended on the grounds that it is professionally irresponsible for a physician to present a therapy as an option to a patient when it "won't work." (8) However, given the current climate of emphasis on patient autonomy, many health care professionals are likely to feel uncomfortable with physicians writing DNR orders without the explicit consent of the patient or his proxy decision maker.

A further difficulty is with the very concept of "futility." The AMA's Council on Ethical and Judicial Affairs has pointed out that "futility" means different things to different people. For example, "some physicians describe a medical treatment as futile only if the possibility of success approaches 0%, whereas others associate futility with success rates as high as 13%." (1) Determinations of futility may be made on the basis of whether the patient survives the initial resuscitation effort. After all, on a purely physiological level, the objective of CPR is to restore cardiac and respiratory function. (1) Futility may also be judged according to length of patient survival; for example, whether the patient survives until she can be discharged from the hospital. (1) Futility might also be defined in terms of the physician's judgment of the quality of life that will be enjoyed by the surviving patient. (1) Yet another definition, which seeks to take account of patient autonomy, suggests that "resuscitative efforts...would be considered futile if they could not be expected to achieve the goals expressed by the informed patient." (1) Thus, the Council on Ethical and Judicial Affairs has suggested that the concept of futility, "which cannot be meaningfully defined," be replaced by "reliance on openly stated ethical principles and acceptable standards of care." (11)

With respect to DNR orders specifically, the Council has taken the following position:

> If, in the judgment of the attending physician, it would be inappropriate to pursue CPR, the attending physician may enter a do-not-resuscitate (DNR) order into the patient's record. Resuscitative efforts should be considered inappropriate by the attending physician only if they cannot be expected either to restore cardiac or respiratory function to the patient or if they meet established ethical criteria.... (12)

The established ethical criteria in question include such factors as likelihood of benefit, change in quality of life, duration of benefit, and the amount of resources required for successful treatment. (13, 14)

In apparent deference to patient autonomy, the Council goes on to recommend, "when there is adequate time to do so, the physician must first inform the patient, or the incompetent patient's surrogate, of the content of the DNR order, as well as the basis for its implementation." (12) Further, "the physician also should be prepared to discuss appropriate alternatives, such as obtaining a second opinion (e.g., consulting a bioethics committee) or arranging for transfer of care to another physician." (12)

In sum, the recommendations of the AMA's Council on Ethical and Judicial Affairs can be seen as trying to strike a balance between the judgment of the physician about appropriate medical treatments and respect for patient autonomy.

Executing and Following DNR Orders

It is appropriate to raise the issue of withholding resuscitation under circumstances such as these:
- The patient is terminally ill.
- The patient has a severe and irreversible illness or disabling condition.
- The patient has suffered an irreversible loss of consciousness.
- The patient is likely to lose decision-making capacity.
- There is likely to be no medical benefit from resuscitation. (15)

Health care facilities typically have policies indicating the procedures to be followed in writing orders to withhold resuscitation. An order to withhold resuscitation must be written by a physician. It is not enough that a patient verbally expresses a desire not to be resuscitated. Ethically, it would be appropriate for health care providers to follow the patient's verbal instructions, but they may be legally bound to provide resuscitation if the written order is not in place. Similarly, an advance directive is not enough in itself to ensure that resuscitation will be withheld; a written order from a physician is still needed. An advance directive may indicate that an individual does not wish to be resuscitated under certain circumstances, but the written physician order is still required. An order to withhold resuscitation is documented in the patient's chart, and is reviewed periodically to see if it is still appropriate.

At one time some health care providers engaged in "slow codes" or "show codes." In these instances staff took their time in responding to a call for resuscitation or otherwise gave the appearance of performing resuscitation while not really making a full effort to do so. Such practices are morally objectionable in being deceptive. They may be explicitly forbidden by a facility's policies.

A DNR order does not automatically mean that no other therapeutic or life-sustaining measures will be given to a patient. A DNR order may be in place while other forms of aggressive treatment are provided.

EMS Personnel and DNR Orders

It has been an issue whether emergency medical services (EMS) personnel should honor a DNR order when called to a home or to provide transportation for a resident. Their job, after all, is to provide emergency medical services in life-threatening situations. This issue is being resolved in favor of EMS personnel honoring DNR orders. (16, 17) Legislatively, there has been a movement to cover precisely this sort of situation for EMS personnel through the establishment of "out-of-hospital DNR orders." Such special DNR orders "apply when a panicked relative calls the rescue squad for a patient under hospice care; when a patient is being transported by ambulance; and potentially in a variety of other public and private settings, such as schools or nursing homes." (18)

FOR GROUP DISCUSSION

1. If you are connected with a long-term care facility, review the facility's DNR policy from an ethical perspective. Does the policy respect the ethical value of patient autonomy? Does it give any recognition to the ethical principle of weighing benefits and burdens in making decisions about resuscitation? Does it contain any stipulations pertaining to "futile" resuscitation attempts? Do you think the policy is in need of revision or refinement in any way?

2. Standards for long-term care developed by the Joint Commission on Accreditation of Healthcare Organizations (JCAHO) include criteria for evaluating a facility's performance with respect to DNR orders. First of all, residents should be involved in decisions to provide or withhold resuscitative services. [RI.2.19] Further, the facility should have in place a framework for a decision-making process that addresses the facility's position on initiating resuscitative services and conflicts regarding provision or withholding of resuscitative services. Further, the governing body of a facility should approve all processes involving resuscitative services, and residents should be informed of the facility's position and policies on resuscitative services at the time of admission. [RI.2.19] (19)

   If you are connected with a long-term care facility, review the facility's DNR practices from the perspective of JCAHO standards.

3. Consider the case of Roger Murray presented above. Suppose you are a member of the ethics committee to which the resident advocate brings this case. Suppose further that the physician in question is asked to attend the meeting at which this case is discussed. (You might have one person role play the part of the resident advocate, other person assume the role of the physician, and yet others take the roles of ethics committee members.)

   • What concerns might be expressed by the resident advocate?

   • What might the physician say in defense of writing a DNR order without the resident's consent?

   • What questions and issues might be raised by members of the ethics committee?

- Should the resident's religious beliefs overrule considerations about the lack of benefit of a treatment from a medical point of view?

- After considering the various points of view, how do you think this situation should have been handled? What factors and ethical principles are important in coming to this judgment?

4. Suppose that a resident, Anne, who has a DNR order, suffers an arrest as a result of choking on food in the dining room. In addition to having the written DNR order on her chart, Anne has repeatedly stated that she "never wants anyone beating on her chest" to resuscitate her. However, her arrest is not due to an underlying disease process that will naturally progress to death, but to an accident. Should CPR be performed on Anne?

Suppose that another resident, Nora, who also has a DNR order, suffers an arrest due to a negative reaction to new medication that her doctor has prescribed for her. Should CPR be performed on Nora?

NOTES

1. Council on Ethical and Judicial Affairs, American Medical Association, "Guidelines for the Appropriate Use of Do-Not-Resuscitate Orders," *Journal of the American Medical Association* 265/14 (April 10, 1991): 1868-71.
2. American Heart Association, "Ethical Considerations in Resuscitation," *Journal of the American Medical Association* 268/16 (Oct. 28, 1992): 2282-88.
3. Steven H. Miles, Robert Koepp, Eileen P. Weber, "Advance End-of-Life Treatment Planning," *Archives of Internal Medicine* 156 (May 27, 1996): 1062-67.
4. Donald J. Murphy, David Burrows, et al., "The Influence of the Probability of Survival on Patients' Preferences Regarding Cardiopulmonary Resuscitation," *New England Journal of Medicine* 330/8 (Feb. 24, 1994): 544-49.
5. HCFA Health Standards and Quality Regional Letter No. 97-10 dated May 9, 1997 on the subject of Provider-wide Blanket "Do Not Resuscitate" Orders.
6. Barbara Springer Edwards, "DNR in the OR?" *American Journal of Nursing* 97/3 (March 1997): 66.
7. Judith O. Margolis, Brian J. McGrath, et al., "Do Not Resuscitate (DNR) Orders During Surgery: Ethical Foundations for Institutional Policies in the United States," *Anesthesia and Analgesia* 80 (1995): 806-9.
8. Tom Tomlinson & Howard Brody, "Futility and the Ethics of Resuscitation," *Journal of the American Medical Association* 264/10 (Sept. 12, 1990): 1276-80.
9. James Drane & John Coulehan, "The Concept of Futility: Patients Do Not Have a Right to Demand Medically Useless Treatment," *Health Progress* 74/10 (Dec. 1993): 28-32.
10. Marcia Angell, "The Case of Helga Wanglie A New Kind of 'Right to Die' Case," *New England Journal of Medicine* 325 (1991): 511-12.
11. Council on Ethical and Judicial Affairs of the American Medical Association, *Current Opinions* 2.035. http://www.ama-assn.org/
12. Council on Ethical and Judicial Affairs of the American Medical Association, *Current Opinions* 2.22. http://www.ama-assn.org/

13. Council on Ethical and Judicial Affairs of the American Medical Association, *Current Opinions* 2.03. http://www.ama-assn.org/

14. Council on Ethical and Judicial Affairs of the American Medical Association, *Current Opinions* 2.095. http://www.ama-assn.org/

15. Diane E. Hoffmann, Philip Boyle & Steven A. Levenson, *Handbook for Nursing Home Ethics Committees* (Washington, DC: American Association of Homes and Services for the Aging, 1995).

16. See, for example, the policy statement from the Ethics Committee, American College of Emergency Physicians, "Ethical Issues of Resuscitation," *Annals of Internal Medicine* 21/10 (October 1992): 1277.

17. See, for example, Emergency Cardiac Care Committee and Subcommittee, "Ethical Considerations in Resuscitation," *Journal of the American Medical Association* 268/16 (Oct. 28, 1992): 2282-88.

18. Nancy M.P. King, *Making Sense of Advance Directives*, rev. ed. (Washington, DC: Georgetown University Press, 1996).

19. Joint Commission on Accreditation of Healthcare Organizations, 2002-2003 *Standards for Long-Term Care* (Oakbrook Terrace, IL: Joint Commission Resources, 2002).

FOR FURTHER STUDY

RESUSCITATION

- *Guidelines on the Termination of Life-Sustaining Treatment and the Care of the Dying: A Report by the Hastings Center* (Briarcliff Manor, NY: Hastings Center, 1987), Part Two-B.

- Cynthia B. Cohen (ed.), *Casebook on the Termination of Life-Sustaining Treatment and the Care of the Dying* (Bloomington, IN: Indiana University Press, 1988), Part II-B, nos. 7 and 8. Case studies with commentary.

- Carol Levine (ed.), *Cases in Bioethics Selections from the Hastings Center Report*, 1st ed. (New York: St. Martin's, 1989), no. 22. Case study with commentary.

FUTILE MEDICAL TREATMENT

- Felicia Ackerman, "The Significance of a Wish," *Hastings Center Report* 21/4 (July-August 1991): 27-29.

- Steven H. Miles, "Informed Demand for 'Non-Beneficial' Medical Treatment," *New England Journal of Medicine* 325/7 (Aug. 15, 1991): 512-15.

- E. Haavi Morreim, "Profoundly Diminished Life The Casualties of Coercion," *Hastings Center Report* 24/1 (1994): 33-42.

- Stephen G. Post, "Medical Futility and the Free Exercise of Religion," *Journal of Law, Medicine & Ethics* 23 (1995): 20-26.

- Lawrence J. Schneiderman, Nancy S. Jecker, and Albert R. Jonsen, "Medical Futility: Its Meaning and Ethical Implications," *Annals of Internal Medicine* 112 (June 15, 1990): 949-54.

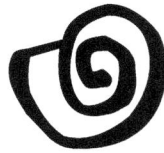

Chapter 10

The Dilemma of Artificial Nutrition and Hydration

After an automobile accident at age 24, Nancy Cruzan entered a persistent vegetative state. She was permanently unconscious, unaware of her surroundings, unable to communicate, and unable to chew or swallow in a normal manner. After four years in this condition in a Missouri hospital, Nancy's family requested that the feeding tube that was keeping her alive be removed and that she be allowed to die. A court order, granting permission to withdraw the feeding tube, was overturned on appeal to the Missouri State Supreme Court. The question of removing Nancy's feeding tube eventually went to the United States Supreme Court. (1) Both legally and ethically, the issue of withholding or withdrawing tube feeding has been so controversial that it deserves special attention among life-sustaining treatments.

Tube feeding, or more technically, *artificial nutrition and hydration*, can take various forms. A needle may be inserted into a vein in the arm; this is known as *peripheral intravenous feeding*. Or a catheter may be inserted into a central vein near the heart, which is called *central intravenous feeding* or *total parenteral feeding* or *hyperalimentation*. Another form is the *nasogastric (NG) tube*, which consists of a thin plastic tube inserted through the nose into the stomach or into the first portion of the duodenum. A *gastrostomy tube* is inserted directly into the stomach, either surgically or through an incision made with the assistance of an endoscope (PEG—percutaneous endoscopic gastrostomy). A *jejunostomy tube* is placed in the small intestine, either surgically or by a method similar to PEG tube placement. (2, 3)

Tube feeding may be used on a short-term basis following surgery when the patient temporarily cannot eat. (2) Such uses of tube feeding are not controversial. But tube feeding can also be used for longer periods of time in a variety of circumstances in which the patient cannot get adequate nutrition and hydration by normal means. A patient may be unable to swallow because of a stroke. An obstruction can occur in the esophagus or pharynx. Cancers can block the gastrointestinal tract. Enzymes necessary to absorb nutrients in the intestines may be inadequate. Or, while the patient may have a normal mouth, stomach, and intestinal tract, she may be averse to or uninterested in eating. An individual suffering from dementia may be unable to remember how to eat or drink and thus no longer swallows. (2, 3) From an ethical point of view, tube feeding has been controversial when used for a prolonged period of time as a means (and sometimes the only means) of continuing to keep a patient alive.

This chapter covers:
* *the controversy whether artificial nutrition and hydration should be classified as "standard nursing care" or as a "medical treatment";*
* *the benefits and burdens of artificial nutrition and hydration;*
* *common misunderstandings about artificial nutrition and hydration;*

- *issues about artificial nutrition and hydration specific to the long-term care setting;*
- *guidelines developed by associations of health care professionals for the provision of artificial nutrition and hydration.*

CASE STUDY

Barbara Ryan, a 60 year-old widow, is the kind of grandmother whose life revolves around her six grandchildren. She is constantly doing things with them and taking them places. Barbara has always enjoyed reasonably good health. Everyone is surprised when she collapses at a church picnic to which she has taken three of her grandchildren.

At the hospital, Barbara's daughter Ann and son Robert are told that Barbara has suffered a stroke. Because of this, she cannot swallow normally. Ann and Robert have no qualms about consenting to the placement of a feeding tube for their mother.

After a week, Barbara is transferred to the Forest Glen Nursing Home. Her family visits her frequently. Because Barbara's grandchildren are anxious for her to get well, Barbara's daughter and son insist that her physician and the nursing home staff do everything necessary for her recovery.

However, Barbara eventually lapses into a semiconscious state. She doesn't recognize family members or friends when they come to visit her. She is bedridden, listless, and suffers periodic bouts with pneumonia.

After their mother has been in this condition for two years, Ann and Robert begin to reassess their directive to the physician and nursing home staff to "do everything" for their mother. They recall a statement she made while taking care of their dying father. She said most emphatically that she was "ready to die when God wanted to take her" and wanted "no heroic measures to interfere with God's plan."

Ann goes to court to be named her mother's legal guardian. With the agreement of her brother, Ann requests that the artificial nutrition and hydration that is keeping their mother alive be stopped. Barbara's physician agrees to this request.

However, the facility's dietitian, Rhonda Pierce, who has been involved in Barbara's care for the past two years, becomes very upset when she hears that Barbara's feeding tube will be removed. She believes it is wrong to deny any person food and water. In fact, Rhonda tells the facility's administrator that, if Barbara's feeding tube is removed, she will have to consider quitting her job because she does not want to be part of a resident being "starved to death."

Artificial Nutrition and Hydration:
"Standard Nursing Care" or "Medical Treatment"

The dietitian in our case believes that it is wrong to deny any person food and water. One issue that arose early in the debate over artificial nutrition and hydration is whether the procedure should be classified as "standard nursing care" and hence should always be provided, or whether it should be regarded as a "medical treatment" to be used or forgone on the same basis as other life-sustaining treatments.

Those who regard tube feeding as standard nursing care have put forward several arguments in support of their view. They point out that, while medical treatment is therapeutic, nutrition and hydration are not because they will not cure a disease. (4, 5) However, in rebuttal it could be said that not all recognized medical treatments cure disease. For example, kidney dialysis does not cure the problem of kidney failure, but simply provides a way of circumventing the problem. Similarly, tube feeding circumvents problems with eating.

It has also been argued that withholding or withdrawing food and fluids is different than withholding or withdrawing medical therapies because of its finality. Withholding or withdrawing food and fluids ensures death, whereas in the case of removing a patient from a ventilator, for example, the patient may surprise us and breathe on her own. (4, 5, 6, 7) However, this line of argument ignores the fact that stopping dialysis inevitably results in a patient's death, as does a decision not to perform cardiopulmonary resuscitation when a cardiac arrest occurs. (8)

Morever, in the case of an unconscious patient a ventilator and a feeding tube are alike in that both replace normal bodily functions that are compromised by that patient's illness. (9)

It should also be kept in mind that some feeding tubes are surgically inserted, and this is certainly a medical procedure. In addition, a feeding tube is used by a physician's order, and is monitored by a physician or someone working under a physician's direction. (9)

In sum, we will regard tube feeding as a medical treatment, as is common practice today. (10) The very terminology "artificial" nutrition and hydration is significant. What we are discussing here is very different from assisting a patient to eat with a spoon.

The Benefits and Burdens of Artificial Nutrition and Hydration

Given that tube feeding is a medical treatment, it should be used or forgone on the same basis as all other life-sustaining treatments. Following the principle of patient autonomy, we need to ask whether the patient herself would want tube feeding in a particular case. And the patient should be encouraged to make her choice by weighing the benefits and burdens of tube feeding. (See the chapter "Making Decisions about Using or Forgoing Life-Sustaining Treatments.")

Tube feeding can benefit patients in several ways. It offers the very fundamental benefit of "prolonging life in patients who are unable to take adequate nutrition by mouth." (11) It can also benefit patients by providing time to treat underlying medical problems or to clarify the patient's prognosis. (11) However, we must be careful not to exaggerate the benefits of artificial nutrition and hydration.

For one thing, there are cases in which tube feeding will not be effective in prolonging life. For example, a patient may be suffering from such severe heart, kidney, or liver failure that that his body cannot process, metabolize, or excrete the nutrients or fluids supplied by a feeding tube. (3) Or again, it may be virtually impossible to attach a feeding tube to a patient with nearly total body burn. (12) When tube feeding would be futile, there is, according to the principle of weighing benefits and burdens, no moral obligation to attempt it.

Tube feedings also carry the burden of involving some physical risks and complications. For example, a needle inserted into a vein in the arm or leg carries the risk of infection, inflammation, and clotting (2) and cannot be used on a long-term basis because the veins will eventually collapse. (13) Tubes inserted into the digestive tract can cause nausea, vomiting, diarrhea, inadequate gastric emptying, and malabsorption, and the reflux of gastric contents can lead to aspiration pneumonia. (14) The retention of a nasogastric feeding tube is uncomfortable and irritating to patients. (2, 13) Nasogastric tubes can press against the lining of the nostrils and pharynx and lead to ulceration. They can also interefere with drainage from the sinuses, leading to blockage and infection. (3)

Gastrostomy and jejunostomy tubes are more comfortable for patients, but surgical insertion carries some risk of infection and bleeding. (2, 13) Use of the PEG procedure for insertion of a gastrostomy tube may result in perforation of the gastrointestinal tract, infection of the abdominal cavity (peritonitis), bleeding, and infection at the site of the tube placement. (3) Use of a jejunostomy tube may cause the patient to have more difficulties with diarrhea. (3)

In addition, there is a problem with angry, confused, or demented patients pulling out nasogastric tubes, with the result that mechanical or chemical restraints are applied to patients to keep the feeding tube in place. (11, 13, 15) Such restraints are surely a burdensome aspect of this procedure for the patient.

In the case of patients who are dying, it has been found that artificial hydration may actually increase their discomfort during their dying process by exacerbating problems with edema, vomiting, and incontinence. Conversely, the natural process of dehydration can make the dying patient more comfortable (see below). (16) The discomfort which artificial hydration can cause a dying patient is likewise a burden to be considered in making a decision about its use in such a case.

What is important to keep in mind is that tube feeding is a mixed blessing. While it can benefit a patient, there are also burdens that can be associated with it. As with all life-sustaining treatments, decisions about using or forgoing artificial nutrition and hydration must be made on a case-by-case basis.

Common Misunderstandings about Artificial Nutrition and Hydration

The dietitian in our case study describes the removal of the feeding tube from Barbara Ryan as "starving a patient to death." We often hear this phrase used in cases where a decision is made to withhold or withdraw tube feeding. But this description involves some misconceptions about forgoing artificial nutrition and hydration.

First, the phrase "starving a patient to death" carries the connotation that we are doing something to cause the patient's death, or engaging in an act of euthanasia.

Second, the description "starving a patient to death" conjures up images of a painful, agonizing death.

One definition of euthanasia is "an action or an omission which of itself or by intention causes death, in order that all suffering may in this way be eliminated." (17) If we are dealing with some underlying fatal pathology that makes the feeding tube necessary in the first place (for example, a stroke which makes the patient unable to swallow), the removal or withholding of the feeding tube merely allows that fatal pathology to take its natural course. It is the underlying fatal pathology, not the absence of the feeding tube, that is the direct cause of death. Further, the intent behind the removal or withholding of the feeding tube is important. If the purpose is to relieve the patient of a procedure that is of limited usefulness or unreasonably burdensome, then this decision can be seen as different than a decision to kill a patient. (13) Thus withholding or withdrawing the feeding tube under these conditions is not an act of euthanasia on our part. (For further explanation of these distinctions, see the chapter "Euthanasia and Assisted Suicide.")

On another level, the description "starving a patient to death" conjures up images of a painful, agonizing death. It is simply not true that a patient who is not given tube feedings will die in this way. For one thing, sensations of hunger and thirst can be relieved without using medical nutrition and hydration procedures. For example, ice chips or glycerin swabbing of the mouth can be used to relieve the thirst of dehydrated patients. (10, 18) Further, there is evidence that patients who are allowed to die without artificial nutrition and hydration may die more comfortably than patients who receive conventional amounts of intravenous hydration. (16) Dehydration can reduce the patient's secretions and excretions, thus relieving breathing problems and decreasing problems with vomiting and incontinence. Indeed, dehydration leads to death in ways that produce a sedative effect on the brain just before death, thus decreasing the need for pain medication. (16, 18) Consider the following actual case:

> David was a 64-year-old man with recurrent metastatic cancer of the larynx and tongue. Before being referred to the hospice program, he had received several years of therapy including surgery, radiation, and chemotherapy. He had massive facial and neck deformity with superimposed edema, which had resulted from treatment and recurrent disease. He had a continuous flow of secretions from the mouth and the tracheostomy site. His severe pain was managed with morphine sulfate, but maintaining his airway was a serious challenge. Although secretions could be removed by suctioning, the growing tumor and increasing edema threatened total airway occlusion.
>
> The patient, who was alert and oriented and had been feeding himself through a gastric tube, then decided to discontinue tube feedings. He lived 27 days after this decision. During that time, his appearance and comfort improved remarkably. Family members noted that the lessening facial edema made him look more like his usual self. The decrease in the neck edema resulted in a patent airway, which consequently eased the patient's breathing. A decrease in oral secretions also greatly added to his

comfort. David remained mentally alert and interacted with his family. His pain was managed with approximately half of the morphine doses previously necessary. His death came quietly and comfortably. (19)

Providing food and water to a patient has been seen by some as a symbol of care and concern for that person. For this reason, they believe that tube feedings should always be provided to those who need it physically. But nutrition and hydration supplied by medical means is not always a good expression of loving care and concern:

> Food and water are certainly significant symbols, but the social experience associated with the giving and receiving of food and water may be equally important. The patient receiving intravenous fluids, lying alone in a hospital bed, is having a much less rewarding experience than the patient in a personalized room being given ice chips by a concerned caregiver. Both are receiving water, but there are few other similarities. (20)

> Finally, what are the social and psychological effects of feeding techniques? With tube feedings, the caregiver may focus more attention on technical aspects, such as positioning the tube and checking the gastric residual, than on the patient. If feeding proceeds smoothly, contact between the patient and caregiver can be minimal. Moreover, the patient has no control over tube feedings except to pull out the tube. In contrast, during hand feedings the caregiver may be more attentive and affectionate, talking with the patient or holding his or her hand. Patients with few other ways of exercising control can still determine the timing, pace, and content of hand feeding. ...Hand feedings that provide inadequate nutrition may meet more of the patient's needs than tube feedings that deliver adequate calories impersonally. The psychosocial effects of feeding techniques are especially important when the goal is supportive care. (15)

In sum, we must keep in mind that medical technologies can never replace personal presence and the "human touch" in caregiving.

Special Challenges for Long-Term Care

In the long-term care setting, issues beyond the medical condition of residents may drive the use of feeding tubes in ways that may not be appropriate.

Many long-term care facilities suffer from a shortage of staff. Since feeding a person with dementia can be very time consuming, some decisions about using feeding tubes may be made because of a lack of staff necessary for hand feeding. (3) This dilemma raises the ethical issue of the fair allocation of scarce resources, in this case, the fair allocation of the time and services of staff among various residents (see the chapter "Allocating Resources in Health Care").

Facility administrators may also feel pressured to push for feeding tubes out of concern that state officials will treat weight loss in residents with punitive sanctions. (3) This situation challenges facilities to take a leadership role in "developing care protocols that emphasize a variety of interventions that make it clear that residents are not neglected and that ordinary means are used to provide nutrition and hydration to persons who, for a variety of reasons, have difficulty eating and drinking." (3)

Guidelines from Professional Associations

Various associations of health care professionals have issued statements about the provision of artificial nutrition and hydration to patients. The American Dietetic Association has developed a position paper on feeding the terminally ill adult. It affirms that "the most powerful ethical principle to consider is the patient's right of self-determination, and concomitantly, that "the patient's informed preference for level of nutritional intervention is paramount." (18) It proposes that "the expected benefits, in contrast to the potential burdens, of non-oral feeding must be evaluated by the health care team and discussed with the patient," and acknowledges that "sometimes the risks, burdens of pain, and discomfort of providing nutrition support substantially outweigh the benefits." (18)

In particular, the American Dietetic Association proposes that it is appropriate to consider forgoing artificial nutrition and hydration when some or all of the following conditions are present:

- Death is imminent, within hours or a few days.

- Artificial nutrition and hydration will probably worsen the condition, symptoms, or pain, such as during shock, when pulmonary edema or diarrhea, vomiting, or aspiration would cause further complications.

- A competent patient has expressed an informed preference not to receive aggressive nutrition support which would be ineffective in improving the quality of life and/or which may be perceived by the patient as undignified, degrading, and physically or emotionally unacceptable.

- If available and legally recognized, written directives such as the "living will" or "durable power of attorney for medical care" may indicate the preference of an incompetent patient. Otherwise, the next of kin or patient appointed surrogate of an incompetent patient should be consulted about the patient's probable preference for the level of nutrition intervention, as well as state law. (18)

A position statement *Foregoing Nutrition and Hydration* from the American Nurses' Association includes the following points:

- Artificial nutrition and hydration should be distinguished from the provision of food and water. ...The provision of nourishment and hydration by artificial means (i.e., through tubes inserted into the stomach, intestine, or blood vessel) is qualitatively different from merely assisting with feeding.

- Like all other intervention, artificially provided hydration and nutrition may or may not be justified. It should be instituted or forgone only after a process of reasoned decision making focused upon estimates of benefits and burdens to the patient. ...The burdens vary with the particulars of the patient, the substances to be delivered, the mode of delivery, and the anticipated outcome. ...As in all other interventions, the anticipated benefits must outweigh the anticipated burdens for the intervention to be justified.

- Outcomes such as weight gain, increased caloric intake or changes in laboratory test results do not themselves serve as adequate justification for this intervention. Such changes, in the absence of any relation to overall well-being of the patient as a person, are not persuasive reasons to begin or continue to provide artificial nutrition or hydration.

- Since competent, reflective adults are generally in the best position to evaluate various harms and benefits to themselves in the context of their own values, life projects, and tolerance of pain, their acceptance or refusal of food and fluid should be respected. ...In cases where a patient is unable to make his wishes known, or is unable to evaluate the benefits and harms of refusing artificial nutrition and hydration, the decision of a surrogate should be relied upon. A surrogate decision maker, preferably designated by the patient, is one who makes decisions in the best interest of the patient and without self interest.

- It is morally, as well as legally, permissible for nurses to honor the refusal of food and fluid by competent patients in their care. ...Advance directives such as living wills or the legal assignment of durable power of attorney are indications of choices and values and should be followed. Thus, advance directives, including those involving artificial nutrition and hydration, should be followed. (21)

These two sets of guidelines are consistent with ethical principles we are using: patient autonomy, the extension of *patient autonomy* through advance directives, and the *principle of weighing benefits and burdens*. (See the chapter "Making Decisions about Using or Forgoing Life-Sustaining Treatments" and the chapter "Advance Directives.")

For further discussion of artificial nutrition and hydration in the case of patients who are permanently unconscious, see the chapter "Caring for Patients in a Persistent Vegetative State."

FOR GROUP DISCUSSION

1. Consider the case of Barbara Ryan presented above. Suppose that the issue of withdrawing her feeding tube is brought to the nursing home's ethics committee. Role play the committee's discussion by designating individuals to represent Barbara's children Ann and Robert, the facility's dietitian Rhonda Pierce, and ethics committee members.

   - What are Ann and Robert likely to say in favor of withdrawing the feeding tube?
   - What is Rhonda Pierce likely to think and feel? What arguments might be made against withdrawing the feeding tube? Do these arguments hold up?
   - What ethical principles should the members of the ethics committee introduce into the discussion? What guidelines from professional associations are relevant to this case?
   - After listening to each point of view and considering the relevant ethical principles and guidelines, can those involved in this ethics consult reach agreement on what should be done?

2. Stephen Redding, 67, has been fighting colon cancer for five years. He has undergone numerous rounds of chemotherapy. Initially, the chemotherapy seemed to stop the growth of the cancer, but in the last five months it has been ineffective. For this reason, Stephen has recently decided to discontinue the treatments. He tells his physician, Dr. Ellen McDonald, that he is "ready to die" and just wants to be kept as comfortable as possible until that time comes. Dr. McDonald assures him that he will receive the best pain management available.

Stephen's condition continues to deteriorate. Because he has become so debilitated and the caregiving demands on his wife have become so great, he is admitted to St. Mary's Care Center under their hospice program. Because of the cancerous growth blocking his intestinal tract, Stephen cannot get adequate nutrition by normal means. Dr. McDonald asks Stephen if he wants a feeding tube placed. Dr. McDonald is honest in telling Stephen that the feeding tube will likely prolong his life—and his suffering—for a few months, at the most. Stephen tells Dr. McDonald that he doesn't want the feeding tube. Several days later, Dr. McDonald again raises the issue of the feeding tube with Stephen, just to be sure that Stephen hasn't changed his mind. Stephen indicates that he has discussed this treatment with his wife, and that she supports him in his decision to refuse the feeding tube. Dr. McDonald does not bring up the issue again. Two weeks later, Stephen dies.

A few days later two certified nursing assistants (CNAs) who had cared for Stephen, Alice Simon and Diane Cook, go to the facility's director of nursing (DON) to express concern that a feeding tube had not been used for Stephen. Alice and Diane say that they can understand withholding a feeding tube from a dying resident who is mentally "out of it" and doesn't know what is going on, but they can't deal with withholding feeding from a resident who is mentally alert and talks to them when they come into the room—even though they know the resident is near death and doesn't say that he is hungry. The director of nursing suggests that Alice and Diane meet with St. Mary's ethics committee to discuss their concerns.

Suppose that you are a member of St. Mary's ethics committee. What do you say to CNAs Alice and Diane? What ethical principles are relevant to this case? What guidelines from professional associations might be of help in discussing this situation?

3. Sid Sheridan, 81, is in the Alzheimer's unit of the Jackson Park Care Center. He is in the advanced stage of the disease, and has "forgotten" how to eat. Although staff can eventually get him to take some food by mouth, it is not all that much and Sid has undergone a significant weight loss in the last month.

The director of nursing, Lisa Lynch, worries that state surveyors will fine the facility for improper care of Sid because of his weight loss. For this reason, she approaches Sid's doctor about placing a feeding tube. The doctor agrees that this should be done. Lisa proceeds to contact Sid's wife, Ann, as next of kin, to obtain her permission for placement of the feeding tube.

Sid never could face up to the diagnosis of Alzheimer's disease, and refused to execute any advance directives giving instructions about future medical treatment. He refused even to discuss his end of life care with anyone, including his wife. Because of this, Ann feels she has no choice but to follow the doctor's advice and have the feeding tube placed.

However, Sid becomes very agitated by the presence of the tube and pulls it out. It is reinserted, but Sid pulls it out again. This happens several times over a period of several days. Lisa Lynch contacts Sid's wife, Ann, about the dilemma that is now faced. Either they must put restraints on Sid so that he will not pull out the feeding tube, or forgo use of the feeding tube altogether.

Intuitively, Ann feels that the feeding tube should not be forced on her husband. However, she confides to Lisa that she just isn't sure what the right thing to do really is. Lisa suggests that Ann meet with the facility's ethics committee to help her work through this difficult decision.

Suppose that you are a member of the Jackson Park Care Center's ethics committee. What ethical principles would you apply to this case? What guidelines from professional associations might be of help in dealing with this situation? What recommendation would you make to Ann Sheridan regarding the feeding tube?

NOTES

1. Gregory E. Pence, *Classic Cases in Medical Ethics,* 2nd ed. (New York: McGraw-Hill, 1995), chap. 1.
2. David Major, M.D., "The Medical Procedures for Providing Food and Water: Indications and Effects" in Joanne Lynn (ed.), *By No Extraordinary Means The Choice to Forgo Life-Sustaining Food and Water* (Bloomington, IN: Indiana University Press, 1986).
3. Myles Sheehan, S.J., M.D., "Feeding Tubes: Sorting Out the Issues," *Health Progress* 82/6 (Nov.-Dec. 2001): 22-7.
4. Gilbert Meilaender, "On Removing Food and Water: Against the Stream," *Hastings Center Report* 14/6 (Dec. 1984): 11-13.
5. New Jersey State Catholic Conference, "Providing Food and Fluids to Severely Brain Damaged Patients," *Origins* 16/32 (Jan. 22, 1987): 582-4.
6. Patrick G. Derr, "Nutrition and Hydration as Elective Therapy: Brophy and Jobes from an Ethical and Historical Perspective," *Issues in Law & Medicine* 2/1 (1986): 25-38.
7. Patrick G. Derr, "Why Food and Fluids Can Never Be Denied," *Hastings Center Report* 16/1 (Feb. 1986): 28-30.
8. Dennis Brodeur, "Is a Decision to Forgo Tube Feeding for Another a Decision to Kill?" *Issues in Law and Medicine* 6/4 (1991): 395-406.
9. American Academy of Neurology, "Position of the American Academy of Neurology on Certain Aspects of the Care and Management of the Pesistent Vegetative State Patient," *Neurology* 39 (Jan. 1989): 125-6, reprinted in James J.

Walter & Thomas A. Shannon (eds.), *Quality of Life The New Medical Dilemma* (New York: Paulist Press, 1990).

10. Hastings Center, *Guidelines on the Termination of Life-Sustaining Treatment and the Care of the Dying* (Briarcliff Manor, NY: Hastings Center, 1987).

11. Bernard Lo & Laurie Dornbrand, "Understanding the Benefits and Burdens of Tube Feedings," *Archives of Internal Medicine* 149/9 (Sept. 1989): 1925-6.

12. Joanne Lynn & James F. Childress, "Must Patients Always Be Given Food and Water?" in Joanne Lynn (ed.), *By No Extraordinary Means The Choice to Forgo Life-Sustaining Food and Water* (Bloomington, IN: Indiana University Press, 1986).

13. Committee for Pro-Life Activities of the National Conference of Catholic Bishops, "Nutrition and Hydration: Moral and Pastoral Reflections," *Origins* 21/44 (April 9, 1992): 705-12.

14. Emma L. Cataldi-Betcher et al., "Complications Occurring during Enteral Nutrition Support: A Prospective Study," *Journal of Parenteral and Enteral Nutrition* 7/6 (1983): 546-52.

15. Bernard Lo & Laurie Dornbrand, "Guiding the Hand that Feeds Caring for the Demented Elderly," *New England Journal of Medicine* 311/6 (Aug. 9, 1984): 402-4.

16. Joyce C. Zerwekh, "The Dehydration Question." *Nursing* 83 (Jan. 1983): 47-51.

17. Vatican Congregation for the Doctrine of the Faith, *Declaration on Euthanasia* (Washington, DC: United States Catholic Conference, 1980).

18. American Dietetic Association, "Position of the American Dietetic Association: Issues in Feeding the Terminally Ill Adult," *Journal of the American Dietetic Association* 92/8 (August 1992): 996-1002.

19. Shirley Ann Smith, "Controversies in Hydrating the Terminally Ill Patient," *Journal of Intravenous Nursing* 20/4 (July/August 1997): 193-200 at 197.

20. Phyllis Schmitz and Merry O'Brien, "Observations on Nutrition and Hydration in Dying Cancer Patients" in Joanne Lynn (ed.), *By No Extraordinary Means The Choice to Forgo Life-Sustaining Food and Water* (Bloomington, IN: Indiana University Press, 1986).

21. American Nurses' Association, *Position Statements Foregoing Nutrition and Hydration* (April 2, 1992). http://www.nursingworld.org/readroom/position/ethics/etnutr.htm

FOR FURTHER STUDY

- Joanne Lynn (ed.), *By No Extraordinary Means The Choice to Forgo Life-Sustaining Food and Water* (Bloomington, IN: Indiana University Press, 1986). This anthology examines the problem of artificial nutrition and hydration from both ethical and legal perspectives. It also includes a section on the use of this technology with particular populations, such as the elderly in long-term care facilities, newborns, and permanently unconscious patients.

- Joanne Lynn and Joan Harrold, *Handbook for Mortals Guidance for People Facing Serious Illness* (New York: Oxford University Press, 1999). Chapter 11, "Forgoing medical treatment," discusses artificial nutrition and hydration, including its use for the dementia patient.

- Hank Dunn, *Hard Choices for Loving People*, 4th ed. (Herndon, VA: A&A Publishers, 2001. P.O. Box 1098, Herndon, VA). Tel. 703-707-0169 Fax 703-707-0174. Dunn has served as chaplain of Hospice of Northern Virginia, Leesburg, Virginia. This booklet is intended to assist patients and family members making difficult decisions about life-sustaining treatments. Chapter Two is on artificial nutrition and hydration. The third edition is available in Spanish.

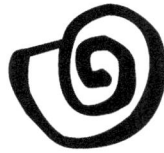

Chapter 11

Treatment Decisions for Persistent Vegetative State (PVS) Patients

Two highly publicized court cases concerning the withdrawal of life-sustaining treatments involved young adult women, Karen Ann Quinlan and Nancy Cruzan. In the case of Karen Ann Quinlan, what was at issue was the removal of a ventilator. In the case of Nancy Cruzan, it was the removal of a feeding tube that proved controversial. What both of these women shared in common was a diagnosis of being in a *persistent vegetative state*. (1)

This chapter covers:
* *medical facts about the persistent vegetative state and related medical conditions;*
* *what the treatment options are for patients in these conditions;*
* *how the principle of patient autonomy and the principle of weighing benefits and burdens apply to treatment decisions for patients in these conditions;*
* *what special ethical issues arise in making treatment decisions for patients in the persistent vegetative state and related medical conditions;*
* *guidelines developed by an association of health care professionals for the provision of artificial nutrition and hydration for such patients.*

CASE STUDY

Don Burns, 35, and Louise Richardson, 32, have been married for six years. They have two children, Jessica, 4, and Eric, 2. All her life Louise has had heart problems because of a congenital heart defect. She feels very fortunate to have been able to carry the two children she now has. Both Don and Louise have established promising careers as attorneys.

Late one afternoon, a neighbor finds Louise lying on the front porch of her home. Apparently, Louise had stopped at home on her way to pick up her children at the day care center when something happened to her. The neighbor calls 911. The paramedics who arrive tell the neighbor that Louise has suffered a cardiac arrest. CPR is administered to restore her heartbeat, and she is taken to the emergency room of the local hospital.

When her husband Don arrives at the hospital, he finds that Louise has been put in the intensive care unit (ICU) and placed on a ventilator. Two weeks go by, and Louise remains "out of it." Sometimes she has roving eye movements, but she doesn't seem aware of anyone in the room. She doesn't speak, and when the doctor tries to get her to respond to simple commands, she doesn't. She is now able to be taken off the ventilator and can breathe on her own, but she must be fed through a tube. A neurologist who examines Louise diagnoses her as being in a "vegetative state."

Louise is transferred to the Woodlands Care Center since there is no special treatment the hospital can provide for her at this point. Her care at the nursing home includes tube feeding, turning her in bed periodically to prevent pressure sores, maintaining appropriate hygiene, and monitoring sugar, protein, and electrolyte levels in her blood.

Three weeks after admission to the Woodlands Care Center—and five weeks after the cardiac arrest which put her in this condition—Louise develops pneumonia. She is again examined by a neurologist, who tells Don that his wife is now in a "persistent vegetative state" and that he will have to make decisions about the kinds of treatments which should and should not be provided for his wife.

Without hesitation, Don insists that antibiotics—and any other treatment medically indicated—be provided for his wife. It is too soon, he believes, to give up on the possibility of his wife's recovery. He himself has seen several cases of patients who were written off as "hopeless" by doctors but who eventually recovered. Besides, he points out that his wife is still very young, only 32 years old—much too young to be allowed to die. Indeed, for the sake of their two young children who need a mother, Don wants "everything possible" done to save Louise.

Two certified nursing assistants (CNAs) at the care center are overhead saying that they are glad Louise's husband made this decision. After all, how could he or the doctors let someone die whose eyes are open?

Medical Facts about PVS

Before considering the ethical issues surrounding care of PVS patients, it is very important to know certain medical facts about this condition. The term "persistent vegetative state" is frequently used generically. More technically, a distinction is now being made between a vegetative state, a *persistent* vegetative state, and a *permanent* vegetative state. (2, 3)

A *vegetative state* is one form of unconsciousness. It is deceptive to observers because the patient goes through sleep-wake cycles so that there are times when the patient's eyes are open. However, there is no indication that the patient is aware of herself or the environment. Some brain functions are still intact either completely or partially, namely, those controlled by the hypothalamus and the brain stem. (2)

A task force on PVS sponsored by five different medical societies (commonly referred to as the "Multi-Society Task Force on PVS") has proposed the following criteria for diagnosing a vegetative state:

- The patient gives no evidence of being aware of self or the environment, and is unable to interact with others.

- The patient gives no evidence of sustained, reproducible, purposeful, or voluntary behavioral responses to stimuli.

- The patient gives no evidence of understanding or using language.

- The patient goes through sleep-wake cycles.
- The brain functions of the hypothalamus and brain stem are sufficiently preserved to allow the patient to survive with medical and nursing care.
- The patient has incontinence of both bowel and bladder.
- Cranial-nerve reflexes (e.g., reaction of the pupils to light, the gag reflex) and spinal reflexes are preserved in varying degrees. (2, 3)

A patient in a vegetative state may occasionally grunt, scream, smile, or shed tears, and show movement of nonparalyzed limbs. Again, this can be deceiving to observers, who mistakenly take this activity as a sign of consciousness. (2, 3)

A vegetative state is different from a coma. In a coma a patient's eyes remain closed, and she appears to be asleep but cannot be aroused. (2, 3) The patient does not go through sleep-wake cycles as happens in the vegetative state. (3)

A *persistent vegetative state* is defined as a vegetative state that has continued for at least one month. It can occur after an acute traumatic brain injury (e.g., an injury due to a car accident) or after an acute nontraumatic brain injury (e.g., cardiac arrest). It can be caused by degenerative or metabolic disorders (e.g., Alzheimer's disease, Parkinson's disease, Huntington's disease) or by developmental malformations in infants and children (e.g., anencephalic infant in whom part of the brain never develops). (2, 3) Sometimes a patient in a persistent vegetative state because of an acute traumatic or nontraumatic brain injury will regain consciousness and abilities to function in various ways, but the probabilities of this happening are not particularly good. (4)

A patient in a persistent vegetative state is said to enter a *permanent vegetative state* when the diagnosis that the condition is irreversible can be established with a high degree of probability, or, in other words, when the chance that the patient will regain consciousness is very, very small. (2, 3) In the case of a traumatic brain injury, a persistent vegetative state can be considered permanent twelve months after the injury in both adults and children. Recovery after this time is very rare, and almost always involves severe disability. If the persistent vegetative state is related to a nontraumatic injury, it can be considered permanent after three months in both adults and children. While recovery does occur after this time period, it is rare and involves moderate or severe disability. (4) Patients who are in a vegetative state due to degenerative or metabolic diseases have no possibility of recovery. (4) In the case of infants and children with brain malformations severe enough to cause a developmental vegetative state, lack of consciousness by the age of six months almost completely precludes the potential for future improvement. (4) In the case of anencephalic infants, it is clear at birth that there is no possibility for recovery because the complete absence of the cerebral cortex of the brain precludes consciousness. (4)

Most patients in a persistent (or permanent) vegetative state who survive for a long time are able to breathe on their own and have a functioning cardiovascular system. (2) Because she is unconscious, a patient in a persistent or permanent vegetative state is not aware of pain. While such a patient may react in certain ways to painful stimuli (e.g., facial movements), she does not "feel" pain in the sense of conscious discomfort. (3, 4, 5, 6)

Because of the severe brain injury necessary to produce the vegetative state, the average life expectancy of such patients is two to five years. (4) However, a very small number of such patients "have survived for more than 15 years...including three patients who survived for more than 17, 37, and 41 years." (4) Reported causes of death for patients in a persistent (or permanent) vegetative state include pulmonary or urinary tract infection, generalized systemic failure, ventilatory failure, and recurrent strokes or tumors. (4)

Treatment Decisions for PVS Patients

A patient in a persistent (or permanent) vegetative state needs various kinds of care:

> Preventive care is foremost. Daily exercises in a range of movements slow the formation of limb contractures, which otherwise become particularly severe in patients in a persistent vegetative state. Daily skin care and frequent repositioning of the patient prevent decubitus ulcers. A tracheostomy may be required to maintain airway patency and prevent aspiration pneumonia. Bladder and bowel care is desirable for hygienic reasons. Since pulmonary and urinary tract infections are common, appropriate monitoring and, if necessary, treatment with antibiotics are required. Placement of nasogastric, gastrostomy, or jejunostomy feeding tubes is usually necessary to maintain adequate nutrition and hydration. (4)

Those responsible for making health care decisions for persistent (and permanent) vegetative state patients are faced with choosing among several possible levels of treatment:

- Continue routine nursing care, but stop all treatments necessary for prolonging life, including artificial nutrition and hydration.

- Continue artificial nutrition and hydration as well as routine nursing care, but do not add any additional procedures or treatments.

- Continue artificial nutrition and hydration as well as routine nursing care, and add procedures or treatments such as the following if they become necessary for prolonging life: antibiotics, simple diagnostic tests, blood or blood product transfusions, transfer to the intensive care unit (ICU), dialysis, chemotherapy for cancer, minor surgery, major surgery, mechanical ventilation, cardiopulmonary resuscitation, organ transplantation. (4, 7)

For example, in the case study above, Louise's husband has decided that he wants everything provided that is needed medically by his wife (e.g., tube feeding, monitoring of blood levels, antibiotics).

A patient who is in a persistent (or permanent) vegetative state is not capable of making decisions, so that a proxy must make decisions on her behalf. The preferred standard for proxy decision making is the *principle of substituted judgment*, which directs the proxy to make treatment decisions in accord with the values and wishes of the patient. This method of proxy decision making is regarded as an extension of *patient autonomy*. (8) However, a patient's own autonomous judgment as well as a proxy's substituted judgment ought to be guided by the *principle of weighing benefits and burdens*. Thus the proxy should ask: How would this patient judge the respective benefits and burdens of a certain treatment administered while in a persistent (or permanent) vegetative state? (See the chapter "Making Decisions about Using or Forgoing Life-Sustaining Treatments.")

Therapies aimed at reversing the persistent vegetative state have not yet been successful. (3, 4) Some would say that the basic purpose of using treatments to prolong the life of a vegetative state patient (e.g., tube feeding, antibiotics) is to enable the patient to survive long enough to recover consciousness and function. This possible recovery is seen as the *benefit* of the life-sustaining treatments. Hence, when a patient is diagnosed as being in a *permanent* vegetative state, the benefit of using life-sustaining treatments is very, very unlikely to occur. According to this point of view, treatment decisions for someone in a *permanent* vegetative state may be different from decisions for someone in a *persistent* vegetative state where recovery is still a possibility. (9)

Consider the case study involving Louise. She has been in a vegetative state for over one month (specifically, for five weeks) so that she can be reliably diagnosed as being in a *persistent* vegetative state. Her condition is due to a nontraumatic injury (viz., a cardiac arrest), and studies indicate that three months must elapse before her vegetative condition can be judged to be *permanent*. However, studies indicate that when a persistent vegetative state is due to a nontraumatic injury, only 11 percent of such patients recover consciousness by three months after the injury. (4)

In Louise's case, there is still some chance (although not great) that life-prolonging treatments will make possible the benefit of recovering consciousness. If Louise's husband believes that she would want to take this chance, then it is appropriate for him to want life-sustaining treatments to be used at the present time. However, if Louise does not wake up but her condition progresses into a *permanent* vegetative state, then assessment about the value of providing treatments may well change.

Further, it should be kept in mind that a patient in a persistent (or permanent) vegetative state sustained by artificial nutrition and hydration could experience problems that qualify as *burdensome* aspects of continued treatment. For example, such patients are susceptible to feeding-tube site infections, incontinence and other bowel and bladder disorders, bedsores, and deformities caused by muscle deterioration and contracture. These are genuine burdens for the patient even if the patient does not consciously experience them. (10)

Not everyone, however, agrees with this analysis of when it is appropriate to cease treatments. Some special ethical questions have arisen about persistent (and permanent) vegetative state patients that we must also explore.

Special Ethical Questions in Treatment Decisions for PVS Patients

One issue in the debate over how to treat patients in a persistent (or permanent) vegetative state is whether such patients should be regarded as *disabled but not dying* or as *terminally ill*. (6, 11, 12, 13) From a moral point of view, this is not a trivial question. The question of withholding or withdrawing a life-sustaining treatment can legitimately be raised only when a fatal pathology is present. For when a fatal disease process is present and a life-sustaining treatment is not used, then it is the disease which is the real cause of death rather than any human action. And the fact that a natural disease process is the cause of death is one factor distinguishing forgoing a life-sustaining treatment from euthanasia. (14; see also the chapter "Euthanasia and Assisted Suicide")

Those who take the position that a patient in a persistent (or permanent) vegetative state is "disabled but not dying" point out that such a patient can often have her life prolonged for months or even years through artificial nutrition and hydration. Hence, we are not dealing with a situation in which inevitable death is imminent. (15)

On the other hand, two types of arguments are offered for classifying a patient in a persistent (or permanent) vegetative state as terminally ill. First, patients in this condition cannot chew and swallow *in the normal manner* because these are *voluntary* activities, and brain damage prevents these patients from engaging in voluntary, purposeful activities. (9) It is possible to hand-feed these patients by placing food at the back of the throat and thus activating the involuntary swallow reflex. However, tube feeding is used with most of these patients because it is safer and more practical. (8) For present purposes, the point to note is that the inability to chew and swallow in a normal manner is proposed as a *fatal pathology*. (14, 16) Second, a persistent (or permanent) vegetative state involves serious damage or malformation in the brain. The brain is the "integrating organ of the entire person" and "severe trauma to the brain...generally causes various medical problems that can accurately be described as pathologies." (17)

In sum, if one judges that the persistent (or permanent) vegetative state is a disability, then all of the concern and help we offer to disabled and handicapped persons should be given to persons in this condition. On the other hand, if one judges that this state involves a fatal pathology and is a terminal condition, then one can be morally justified in deciding to forgo life-sustaining treatments for such patients.

Another issue in the debate over how to treat patients in a persistent (or permanent) vegetative state is the value of prolonging life on a merely biological level. While certain bodily functions are retained, such patients have lost consciousness and all the accompanying abilities which, most of all, seem to make us human:

> Most of what makes someone a distinctive individual is lost when the person is unconscious, especially if he or she will always remain so. Personality, memory, purposive action, social interaction, sentience, thought, and even emotional states are gone. Only vegetative functions

and reflexes persist. If food is supplied, the digestive system functions and uncontrolled evacuation occurs; the kidneys produce urine; the heart, lungs, and blood vessels continue to move air and blood; and nutrients are distributed in the body. (18)

It is a matter of debate whether the prolongation of mere biological function is a benefit to a person, and a benefit sufficient to justify the use of life-sustaining treatments. Some argue that "human bodily life is a great good" and in fact that "such life is inherently good, not merely instrumental to other goods." (12) Others contend that medicine is about "human wholeness," a wholeness which "means a certain well-working of the enlivened body and its unimpaired powers to sense, think, feel, desire, move, and maintain itself... ." (14)

In sum, if one believes that biological life is valuable in and of itself, then one will likely regard life-sustaining treatments as providing a benefit even to patients in a permanent vegetative state. On the other hand, if one believes that it is mental activities which are most truly human and that bodily health is a means to this end, then one is not likely to see the use of life-sustaining treatments as beneficial to such patients.

Our medical resources are limited. Another issue that has arisen in the care of patients in a persistent (and especially, those in a permanent) vegetative state concerns the allocation of medical resources. As a society, should we use our medical resources to sustain the lives of such patients when these same resources could be used for other patients who would benefit more? This question was raised (and answered in the negative) by a presidential commission on bioethical issues:

> An irresponsible stewardship of society's resources can occur when a permanently unconscious patient is given care that precludes the treatment of others who would be helped far more than the unconscious patient. This could occur, for example, were another patient to receive less beneficial therapy because a scarce support system is being used with a permanently unconscious patient. Whenever there is reason to believe this is happening, the patient with a remediable illness or even a chance of regaining consciousness should be put on the support system even if it precipitates the death of the permanently unconscious patient...

> A second failure of responsible stewardship occurs when resources are expended so lavishly in the care of patients who will never regain consciousness that other important social goals are thwarted....since it is ethically acceptable to limit the provision of treatment, especially when it can at best offer a very small benefit to the patient, policymakers in public and private health care payment programs may legitimately consider means of limiting, or even proscribing, these expenditures. (18)

Ethically, this issue involves distributive justice, that is, fairness in the distribution of benefits and resources. The value one places (or does not place) on sustaining life on a purely biological level will affect how one judges the use of medical resources for persistent (and permanent) vegetative state patients (and whether one disagrees or agrees with the recommendations of the presidential commission).

Because food is so basic to life, withholding or withdrawing tube feeding has, in general, been very controversial. In fact, the issue of withdrawing a feeding tube from a patient in a persistent (or, more accurately, a permanent) vegetative state has resulted in a legal case being taken all the way to the United States Supreme Court. (See the chapter "The Dilemma of Artificial Nutrition and Hydration.")

When artificial nutrition and hydration are withdrawn, patients in a persistent (or permanent) vegetative state usually die within ten to fourteen days. Dehydration and electrolyte imbalance, rather than malnutrition, are the immediate cause of death. Except for dryness of the skin and mucous membranes, it is not readily apparent to family members that the patient is dying of dehydration. Further, appropriate nursing care can prevent these signs of dehydration.

Facial swelling can occur as a result of prolonged administration of artificial nutrition and hydration. But as the patient becomes dehydrated, this swelling decreases and facial features may assume a more normal appearance during the last few days of life. (4) Some fear that allowing persistent (or permanent) vegetative state patients to die in this way is condemning them to an excruciatingly painful death. But it should be kept in mind that such patients are no longer capable of experiencing sensations of hunger or thirst or of experiencing discomfort or pain.

Guidelines from a Professional Association

Following the report of the Multi-Society Task Force on PVS, the American Dietetic Association (ADA) formulated guidelines for feeding a patient in a PVS:

- Feeding should start for a patient in a coma or an unconscious state as soon as he or she is medically stable and should continue at least until a diagnosis of PVS is established.

- Feeding should only be stopped after the patient is diagnosed as permanently unconscious and there is evidence of the patient's wish to stop nutrition and hydration. (8)

It should be noted that there are two conditions placed on stopping artificial nutrition and hydration. In addition to the state of unconsciousness being diagnosed as permanent, it must be the case that the patient himself would not want nutrition and hydration in such a condition. The second condition is emphasized in the ADA's position paper:

> Guidelines for feeding a permanently unconscious patient support the patient's right to self-determination as the overriding principle. Within American society, the individual's right to self-determination generally takes precedence over the beliefs or wishes of health care providers. (8)

> The patient's expressed desire is the primary guide for determining the extent of nutrition and hydration once the patient is diagnosed as being in a PVS. (8)

From an ethical point of view, the American Dietetic Association is placing a premium on patient autonomy.

FOR GROUP DISCUSSION

Suppose that you are a member of the ethics committee of the Woodlands Care Center and that the following cases involving persistent or permanent vegetative state patients are brought to the committee for an ethics consult. In making a recommendation for care, the following options are available:

- Continue routine nursing care, but stop all treatments necessary for prolonging life, including artificial nutrition and hydration.

- Continue artificial nutrition and hydration as well as routine nursing care, but do not add any additional procedures or treatments.

- Continue artificial nutrition and hydration as well as routine nursing care, and add (some or all of) such treatments as the following if they become necessary for prolonging life: antibiotics, simple diagnostic tests, blood or blood product transfusions, transfer to the intensive care unit, dialysis, chemotherapy for cancer, minor surgery, major surgery, mechanical ventilation, cardiopulmonary resuscitation, organ transplantation.

- Other (describe).

In each case, what would you personally recommend as the best course of action? What facts about the case and what ethical principles are important in choosing that course of action? As a group, can you reach agreement about what ought to be done in each case?

1. Patricia Walker, 55, has been diagnosed as being in a permanent vegetative state. Since she became unconscious after a car accident fifteen months ago, Patricia has been on tube feeding. Recently she has developed pneumonia. Patricia's physician, Dr. Eileen Swanson, speaks with her husband, Ralph, and recommends against the use of antibiotics. Indeed, Dr. Swanson mentions to Ralph that perhaps it is time to think about removing the feeding tube as well. Ralph, however, insists that the doctor "do everything" to save his wife. Ralph admits that, after the death of her father, Patricia had stated quite clearly that she herself wanted to "go quickly" and did not wish to linger on for several years in a debilitated state, as had happened to her father. Nevertheless, Ralph says that "miracles can always happen," and that he just doesn't feel right about "giving up" on Patricia at this point. Ralph says he would feel guilty that he would be doing something to "kill" his wife in consenting to withdrawal of the feeding tube. Because Dr. Swanson is concerned that Ralph has false hopes for his wife, she encourages him to meet with the facility's ethics committee to talk about the situation.

2. Consider again the case of Patricia Walker, with the following change of circumstances: Ralph relates that, after the death of her father, Patricia had stated quite clearly that, if anything happened to her so that she could not

take care of herself, she did not want anything done to shorten or prematurely take her life, as she believed had happened to her father while in the hospital.

3. Two months ago Richard McGann, 45, suffered a serious brain injury in a car accident. Since that time he has been unconscious, and a neurologist has told his wife, Alice, that he is in a persistent vegetative state. Tube feeding has been used during this time to sustain his life. Richard has recently developed kidney problems, and Alice must now make a decision about dialysis. Richard had always been very active physically, golfing, bowling, and taking long bicycle rides on nature trails. Because of this, Alice feels that Richard would never want to continue to exist in an unconscious state, confined to bed, and not able to do any of the things he enjoyed about life. Kidney failure, Alice believes, may be a blessing in disguise, "letting her husband go free." Alice tells her husband's doctor that dialysis should not be started. However, because this decision will ensure that Richard will die, the doctor encourages Alice to talk with the facility's ethics committee before she makes the final decision.

NOTES

1. Gregory E. Pence, *Classic Cases in Medical Ethics*, 2nd ed. (New York: McGraw-Hill, 1995).
2. The Multi-Society Task Force on PVS, "Medical Aspects of the Persistent Vegetative State," Part One, *New England Journal of Medicine* 330/21 (May 26, 1994):1499-1508.
3. American Neurological Association Committee on Ethical Affairs, "Persistent Vegetative State: Report of the American Neurological Association Committee on Ethical Affairs," *Annals of Neurology* 33/4 (April 1993): 386-90.
4. Multi-Society Task Force on PVS, "Medical Aspects of the Persistent Vegetative State," Part Two, *New England Journal of Medicine* 330/22 (June 2, 1994): 1572-79.
5. Ronald E. Cranford, "The Persistent Vegetative State: The Medical Reality (Getting the Facts Straight)," *The Hastings Center Report* (Feb./March 1988): 27-32.
6. Bishops of Pennsylvania, "Nutrition and Hydration: Moral Considerations," *Origins* 21/34 (Jan. 30, 1992): 541, 543-53.
7. Ellen Fox and Carol Stocking, "Ethics Consultants' Recommendations for Life-Prolonging Treatment of Patients in a Persistent Vegetative State," *Journal of the American Medical Association* 270/21 (Dec. 1, 1993): 2578-82.
8. American Dietetic Association, "Position of The American Dietetic Association: Legal and Ethical Issues in Feeding Permanently Unconscious Patients," *Journal of the American Dietetic Association* 95/2 (Feb. 1995): 231-4.
9. American Academy of Neurology, "Position of the American Academy of Neurology on Certain Aspects of the Care and Management of the Persistent Vegetative State Patient," *Neurology* 39 (Jan. 1989): 125-6, reprinted in James J. Walter & Thomas A. Shannon (eds.), *Quality of Life The New Medical Dilemma* (New York: Paulist Press, 1990).

10. Michael R. Panicola, "Withdrawing Nutrition and Hydration," *Health Progress* 82/6 (Nov.-Dec. 2001): 28-33.

11. Bishop James McHugh, "Comments After Nancy Cruzan's Death," *Origins* 20/32 (Jan. 17, 1991): 518-19.

12. William E. May et al., "Feeding and Hydrating the Permanently Unconscious and Other Vulnerable Persons," *Issues in Law and Medicine* 3/3 (Winter 1987): 203-11.

13. Texas Catholic Bishops and the Texas Conference of Catholic Health Facilities, "On Withdrawing Artificial Nutrition and Hydration," *Origins* 20/4 (June 7, 1990): 53-5.

14. Kevin O'Rourke, O.P., "Should Nutrition and Hydration Be Provided to Permanently Unconscious and Other Mentally Disabled Persons?" *Issues in Law and Medicine* 5/2 (1989): 181-96.

15. Committee for Pro-Life Activities of the National Conference of Catholic Bishops, "Nutrition and Hydration: Moral and Pastoral Reflections," *Origins* 21/44 (April 9, 1992): 705-12.

16. Kevin O'Rourke, "Open Letter to Bishop McHugh on Hydration and Nutrition," *Origins* 19/21 (Oct. 26, 1989): 351-2.

17. Dennis Brodeur, "Is a Decision to Forgo Tube Feeding for Another a Decision to Kill?" *Issues in Law and Medicine* 6/4 (1991): 395-406.

18. President's Commission for the Study of Ethical Problems in Medicine and Biomedical and Behavioral Research, *Deciding to Forego Life-Sustaining Treatment* (March 1983; reprint New York: Concern for Dying).

FOR FURTHER STUDY

- Gregory E. Pence, *Classic Cases in Medical Ethics   Accounts of Cases That Have Shaped Medical Ethics, with Philosophical, Legal, and Historical Backgrounds*, 2nd ed. (New York: McGraw-Hill, 1995), Chapter 1, "Coma: Karen Quinlan and Nancy Cruzan."

- James J. Walter and Thomas A. Shannon (eds.), *Quality of Life   The New Medical Dilemma* (New York: Paulist Press, 1990). Relevant readings include "Position of the American Academy of Neurology on Certain Aspects of the Care and Management of the Persistent Vegetative State Patient"; William May et al., "Feeding and Hydrating the Permanently Unconscious and Other Vulnerable Persons"; Thomas A. Shannon and James J. Walter, "The PVS Patient and the Forgoing/Withdrawing of Medical Nutrition and Hydration"; President's Commission, "Patients with Permanent Loss of Consciousness"; New Jersey Catholic Conference, "Providing Food and Fluids to Severely Brain Damaged Patients."

- Robert N. Wennberg, *Terminal Choices Euthanasia, Suicide, and the Right to Die* (Grand Rapids, MI: Eerdmans, 1989). Chapter 6 "The Permanently Unconscious Patient." Wennberg approaches the question of care for the permanently unconscious patient from a religious perspective. He argues that what is of special value about human life is personal consciousness because this is what makes it possible for the individual to participate in God's creative and redemptive purposes for human beings. Where there is only biological or bodily human life, that special value no longer attaches to the individual, and consequently, it is legitimate to allow bodily death to proceed unimpeded.

• Robert V. Rakestraw, "The Persistent Vegetative State and the Withdrawal of Nutrition and Hydration," *Journal of the Evangelical Theology Society* 35/3 (Sept. 1992): 389-405. Rakestraw likewise attempts to bring distinctively religious perspectives to bear on the issue of care for the PVS patient. Using the theological concept of a human as an "image of God," Rakestraw defines a human person as "a unique individual, made as God's image, known and cared for by God at every stage of life, with the actual ability or potential to be aware of oneself and to relate in some way to one's environment, to other human beings, and to God." Since the life of a "person" ends when this ability or potential ceases, the PVS patient is dead from a theological point of view, and hence, the discontinuance of nutrition and hydration is justified.

• Donal P. O'Mathuna, "Responding to Patients in the Persistent Vegetative State," *Philosophia Christi* 19/2 (Fall 1996): 55-83. This is a critical response to Rakestraw's paper which also takes issue with the accuracy of the report of the Multi-Society Task Force on PVS.

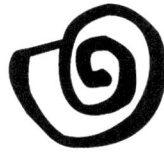

Chapter 12

Advance Directives

An *advance directive* is a document in which an individual makes provision for future medical treatment decisions in the event that he or she loses decision-making capacity. In terms of legal documents, there are two basic types of advance directive: the *living will* and the *durable power of attorney for health care*. These documents may be called by various names in different states.

Advance directives were developed as a way of extending the ethical value of autonomy, that is, self-determination. They allow an individual to control medical treatment decision making when he no longer has the ability to state his wishes directly. Advance directives are also seen as a way of preventing the *overuse* of life-sustaining treatments. People have seen the lives of family members and friends prolonged in a very debilitated state, and their response is —"I would never want that to happen to me!"

This chapter covers:
- *what a living will says and when it goes into effect;*
- *what a durable power of attorney for health care does and how it differs from a living will;*
- *how to execute advance directives;*
- *what requirements for advance directives are set by federal law;*
- *the advantages of having advance directives;*
- *problems with advance directives;*
- *types of advance care planning other than legal advance directives.*

At the present time there is no federal legislation establishing the living will and the durable power of attorney for health care throughout the United States, or establishing a single *form* for executing them. These documents are legally established by the individual states. Nevertheless, all of them share certain features in common.

CASE STUDY

Ted Reed taught math for twenty years at Elkader Community College before retiring two years ago. Since his retirement, Ted has remained so active that his friends from the college joke that he has "flunked retirement." Ted is an avid reader, checking out a new set of books from the library every week. He has resumed playing the piano, something he had to give up because of the time demands of his job. He is a regular volunteer at the local senior center, and continues to tutor students in math at the college. During the summer, he travels around the country attending Elderhostel programs.

Recently, Jim Parker, Ted's friend who also taught math at the college, was diagnosed with cancer. Over a period of a year, Ted visits Jim twice a week. Ted watches Jim suffer from chemotherapy treatments and undergo repeated hospitalizations. His weight loss is significant. At Jim's funeral, Ted comments that Jim doesn't even "look like himself" any more.

Jim's death causes Ted to wonder what would happen if he should be diagnosed with a terminal illness. As far as he is concerned, there would be no point in living if he couldn't continue all the activities that "give his life meaning."

In order to protect himself from ever becoming a "vegetable in a bed," Ted decides to make out advance directives—both a living will and a durable power of attorney for health care document. Ted never married, but he has two sisters and a younger brother. Ted names his brother as his proxy decision maker in executing his advance directives.

One Sunday morning while attending church services, Ted begins to experience severe chest pains. He is taken to the emergency room of the local hospital, where he is diagnosed as having suffered a severe heart attack. Indeed, the doctors in the ER are surprised that Ted has survived at all. After a week in the hospital, Ted is sent to the Elkader Lutheran Home to continue his recuperation.

After three weeks at the Lutheran Home, Ted develops pneumonia. Ted's physician, Dr. Reynolds, thinks Ted should be transferred to the hospital and put on a ventilator to assist his breathing until antibiotics can clear up the pneumonia. Medications being administered to Ted for his heart condition have left him mentally disoriented, and Dr. Reynolds does not think he has the capacity at this point to make sound decisions about his health care. For this reason, Dr. Reynolds contacts Ted's brother to authorize the hospitalization and treatment.

To Dr. Reynolds's surprise, his brother produces Ted's advance directive and says that nothing should be done for Ted's pneumonia. "Ted would never want to live like this," his brother states, "where he can no longer do anything that he used to enjoy." The pneumonia, his brother announces, "is nature's way of granting Ted's wish to die under these circumstances."

Dr. Reynolds disagrees with Ted's brother. In fact, Dr. Reynolds has reservations about the whole idea of advance directives. Living wills, in Dr. Reynolds's view, are too general and vague in the directions they give. The only thing they talk about is forgoing treatment at the very end of the dying process. Moreover, living wills are usually made out by people when they are healthy, and Dr. Reynolds wonders how people can really know what they will want done in situations of serious illness that they have never experienced. When a patient is actually looking death in the face, he may judge holding on to life very differently.

Besides, Dr. Reynolds does not think that Ted is "at the brink of death." He thinks Ted is likely to recover from this bout with pneumonia if it is properly treated. To be sure, Ted's heart problems will leave him with a much restricted life style, but that is not the same as being terminally ill.

Ted's two sisters are also present during the discussion with Dr. Reynolds. They, too, disagree with the judgment of Ted's brother. At this point, they feel everything possible should be done to save Ted's life.

Pastor Susan Wright, who has recently become chaplain at the Lutheran Home, is approached by the facility's administrator about mediating this dispute. She's heard about conflicts that can occur between physicians and family members over treatment decisions. This is the first time that she has witnessed a conflict where a patient's very life is at stake. She herself wonders who is right.

The Living Will

The first type of advance directive developed is the living will. An example of a living will form is included in Appendix 1 of this chapter.

A living will typically goes into effect when a person is suffering from *an incurable or irreversible disease* and is *expected to die within a short period of time*. In some states, the condition of permanent unconsciousness is also included in the scope of the living will. A living will basically says that the individual does not want life-sustaining treatments used in these circumstances. In such cases, life-sustaining treatments would not help improve the person's condition but would only prolong the dying process. However, comfort care and pain medication will still be provided to the individual.

Some people are afraid to sign a living will because they think they will automatically be denied treatment in the case of any medical emergency. This is not true. A living will goes into effect only when the person's illness is incurable or irreversible and death is imminent (or when the person has been reliably diagnosed to be in a state of permanent unconsciousness). For example, if someone with a living will is in a car accident and is taken to the hospital emergency room and can recover, this document will not prevent her from receiving treatment to aid in the recovery.

It is very important to keep in mind *when* a living will goes into effect. For example, in the case scenario about Ted, the physician believes it would be a mistake to forgo aggressive treatment at this point because Ted is not "at the brink of death," and because living with restrictions is not the same as being "terminally ill." In other words, the physician is questioning whether the living will document has really become applicable in Ted's case.

It is also important to keep in mind that a living will goes into effect only when an individual no longer has the capacity to make his own decisions. If someone is in the final stages of the dying process but is conscious and lucid, he should still be asked directly what he does and does not want done in terms of medical treatments.

Durable Power of Attorney for Health Care

Because of limitations in the living will, another form of advance directive has been developed, namely, the durable power of attorney for health care. An example of a form for this document is included in Appendix 2 of this chapter.

The language of a living will document usually gives only general directives about life-sustaining treatments. When signing such a document, an individual cannot foresee all the particular conditions that will prevail when the use of life-sustaining treatments becomes an issue in his own case. Indeed, in the case scenario about Ted, the physician voices the opinion that living wills are too vague...to be of much help in determining what treatments a patient would want. In order to provide for better decision making, a durable power of attorney for health care allows an individual to designate legally someone to make treatment decisions on his behalf when he is no longer able to do so. The legally designated proxy can engage in give-and-take discussion of medical alternatives.

The proxy should be someone who knows well the person's values and preferences, and who can accurately predict what he or she would want done. Indeed, it is the proxy's job *to represent that individual's point of view*, not to make decisions on the basis of what he personally thinks is best. The proxy may be (and often is) a relative, but need not be. It may also be possible to designate someone as an *alternate* proxy should the designated proxy be unavailable at the time a treatment decision must be made.

The durable power of attorney for health care is broader in scope than a living will. It goes into effect in any situation in which the person in question becomes incapable of making treatment decisions. It is not limited to cases in which death is imminent (or the person is permanently unconscious). For example, suppose that someone—let's call him Robert—has executed this document naming his wife Elaine as his legal proxy. And suppose that Robert gets into a car accident, suffers a concussion and broken ribs, and is taken to the hospital unconscious. Elaine will have the legal authority to make any needed treatment decisions on Robert's behalf. And when Robert regains consciousness and decision-making capacity, the right to make treatment decisions will go back to him.

The individual designated as the proxy decision maker through a durable power of attorney for health care *legally* has the right to make treatment decisions and even takes precedence over relatives of the patient or resident. Many families are not aware of this. For example, in the case scenario about Ted, Ted's sisters want the physician to do whatever is necessary to save Ted's life while his brother wants only comfort care given. It is his brother whom Ted chose as his proxy decision maker in executing a durable power of attorney for health care. Hence, it is his brother who has the right to make the treatment decision, not Ted's sisters. Ted's brother may surely consult with his sisters, but legally he has the final say about what happens.

It is also important to keep in mind that a durable power of attorney for health care is a different legal document than a power of attorney for financial matters. The individual designated to take care of someone else's finances does not automatically have the power to make medical decisions for that person.

Executing Advance Directives

It is not absolutely necessary to see a lawyer to execute a living will or durable power of attorney for health care. Health care facilities have individuals on staff trained to provide assistance in making out these documents.

At the present time there is no federal legislation establishing the living will and durable power of attorney for health care for the entire United States, or establishing a standard form for executing them. Legally, these documents have been established state by state. Basically, the content of them is the same, but there may be differences among various states on such matters as who may witness the document, notarization rather than witnessing, or restrictions on who may be named as the proxy decision maker. The documents may also include spaces to write in directions about specific treatments that are or are not wanted (e.g, resuscitation, dialysis, chemotherapy). In some states individuals may be required to give explicit directions about artificial nutrition and hydration or about treatment in a condition of permanent unconsciousness.

Thus the question arises of whether an advance directive written in one state will be recognized in other states. The Commission on Legal Problems of the Elderly of the American Bar Association has given this response:

> Many states expressly recognize out-of-state advance directives if the directive meets either the legal requirements of the state where executed or the state where the treatment decision arises. Several states are silent on this question. If there is doubt, the rules of the state where treatment takes place, not the state where the advance directive was signed, will normally control. (1)

The Commission advises that "even if an advance directive fails to meet technicalities of state law, health providers still should value the directive as important, if not controlling, evidence of the patient's wishes." (1)

While the original of an advance directive should be kept in a safe place, advance directives are not meant to be hidden. Copies of advance directives should be given to the person's physician, family members, and proxy decision maker. The provisions of these documents should be discussed with them so that they feel comfortable with the instructions about treatment. It is also good to give a copy of advance directives to the hospital the person uses to have on record in the event of admission. Copies should also be provided to other health care facilities and services the person is using (for example, a nursing home or hospice program). It may also be a good idea to give copies to close friends and neighbors, since these are sometimes the first individuals to find someone at home undergoing a health care crisis. Some people also keep a reduced size photocopy of their advance directives in their wallets.

Advance directives are not just for senior citizens. They may be executed by anyone who has reached the legal age of adulthood and is mentally competent. They are useful for any adult to have. In fact, two well-known court cases about the withdrawal of life-sustaining treatments, namely, the cases of Karen Ann Quinlan and Nancy Cruzan, involved young adults in their twenties and thirties!

Advance directive documents can be changed or even revoked. They should be reviewed periodically to ensure that they still reflect the wishes of the person who has executed them.

The Patient Self-Determination Act

Federal legislation, called the *Patient Self-Determination Act*, has established requirements regarding advance directives for health care providers receiving Medicare and/or Medicaid funding. Specifically, the legislation sets the following requirements:

- A health care facility or agency must provide written information to each adult concerning his or her rights under state law to make decisions concerning medical care. This should include information about the right to accept or refuse medical or surgical treatment and the right to formulate advance directives.

- A health care facility or service must have written policies respecting the implementation of these rights.

- A health care facility or service must inquire in the case of each adult whether she has an advance directive.

- Documentation must be made in the patient's medical record whether he has executed an advance directive.

- A health care facility or service cannot condition the provision of care or otherwise discriminate against an individual based on whether she has executed an advance directive.

- A health care facility or service must comply with the requirements of state laws respecting advance directives.

- Health care facilities and services must provide education on advance directives for staff and for the community at large. (2)

The law does *not* require a health care facility or agency to carry out any directive whatever contained in a living will or durable power of attorney for health care. No facility or agency is required to act contrary to its mission and ethical values, even if a patient requests this in writing. However, a facility or service must provide written policies specifying the limits on the procedures it will perform. And a clear summary of the facility's or service's policies regarding advance directives and consent to or refusal of medical treatment must be available to the public. (2)

It is very important to recognize that the Patient Self-Determination Act does not require anyone to execute advance directives, but only requires that patients be informed that these documents are available for their use.

Finally, health care workers may be required to attend in-service programs on advance directives. Such educational programs for the staff of a health care facility or service are mandated by the Patient Self-Determination Act. (2)

Advantages of Advance Directives

Autonomy (self-determination) is a value much emphasized in health care today. Advance directives are a useful tool for health care providers in learning what an

---

individual does and does not want done when the person is no longer able to express her wishes directly. They are especially important documents in the long-term care setting because of the incidence of dementia among residents.

Health care providers may sometimes be reluctant to withhold or withdraw life-sustaining treatments for fear of being legally liable. However, if an advance directive has been executed and the health care provider acts in accord with it in not providing life-sustaining treatments, the health care provider has protection. (3) Thus, advance directives can make health care providers more comfortable about complying with requests to forgo life-sustaining treatments.

Advance directives can also be useful when conflicts arise among family members or between family members and health care providers. In such circumstances, if a durable power of attorney for health care has been executed, the designated proxy legally has the power to make the final decision and bring the conflict to resolution. The statements contained in an advance directive can be taken as good evidence of an individual's wishes regarding treatments. Executing advance directives can prevent conflicts from going to court for resolution.

Problems with Advance Directives

In the case scenario at the beginning of this chapter, the physician expresses the opinion that living wills represent decisions made by people in healthy situations and that they should not be recognized in a medical situation that a patient has never previously experienced. The physician is stating one reservation that has been voiced about advance directives. When a person is healthy and active, he may view life with a serious, debilitating illness as unacceptable. But when he is actually in such a condition, holding on to life may appear very different. (For example, what is your own reaction right now to the possibility of suffering an accident that would leave you a quadriplegic in a wheelchair? And might you change your mind if this actually happened to you?)

In sum, executing an advance directive requires an individual to project what he would and would not want done in types of health situations he may never have experienced. But can anyone accurately predict how he will *feel* in such circumstances?

Or consider a related problem. Let's suppose that Jack, aged 66, has prepared advance directives stipulating that "under no circumstances" does he want to be hooked up to a breathing machine "for any illness." And let's further suppose that Jack subsequently is suffering from delirium and Guillan-Barré syndrome, a potentially reversible illness causing progressive weakness and paralysis. Jack's physician recommends to his wife, Thelma, that he be placed on a ventilator, telling her that there is a 60 percent chance of full recovery with temporary mechanical support. Thelma knows the instructions Jack gave in his advance directives. She also believes that, when Jack gave these instructions, he thought that being connected to a ventilator meant only that he would be a "vegetable" with no chance of recovery. She thinks that if Jack knew he had a chance of recovery by being placed on a ventilator, he would take it. (4)

This case illustrates the point that, in making out an advance directive, an individual cannot envision all the possible types of circumstances he might be in. Anyone executing an advance directive needs to be careful to allow some room for discretionary judgment, and not make instructions so specific or absolute as to preclude medically beneficial treatment.

There are several problems health care providers may encounter in using advance directives. For one thing, patients may say they have these documents but forget to bring them to the health care facility or service so that they can be placed in the medical record and actually guide treatment decision making. Or again, it may not be understood that an advance directive is *not* the same thing as a Do-Not-Resuscitate Order, which must be written by a physician (see the chapter "Resuscitation"). Another common problem is that family members do not understand the legal status of the proxy decision maker named through a durable power of attorney for health care, namely, that this individual has the final say in medical treatment decision making and takes precedence over any relative. This lack of understanding can result in family conflict. Or again, it may be unclear whether an individual still has the mental competency to make medical treatment decisions and, concomitantly, it will be unclear whether an advance directive should become operative.

The durable power of attorney for health care carries its own special problems. It is not unusual for an individual to ask a family member to serve as her proxy decision maker. However, it may be emotionally difficult for this family member to make a decision to "let go" of a loved one by forgoing life-sustaining treatments, even though this is what the individual in question would have wanted. In other words, acting as a proxy decision maker for medical treatments can prove a burdensome task to assume. (3)

Further, residents of advanced age in long-term care facilities may have outlived the family members and friends who would be candidates for selection as their proxy decision maker. And if they have no one to designate to serve in this capacity, they are precluded from executing this type of advance directive. (3)

Other Types of Advance Care Planning

A living will or a durable power of attorney for health care can only be executed by someone who is mentally competent. Thus, if someone is suffering from dementia and has not already executed an advance directive, he can no longer do so. Similarly, persons who have suffered from severe mental retardation since birth cannot execute advance directives.

A person can only execute an advance directive for himself or herself. So, for example, a parent cannot execute an advance directive for a young adult son or daughter who is mentally retarded. A wife cannot execute an advance directive for a husband suffering from dementia. In such cases a decision may be made to ask the court to officially appoint a *guardian* to make treatment decisions for the patient, or often family members close to the patient simply make such decisions. Some health care facilities have forms family members may fill out to indicate types of treatments that should and should not be administered. While such documents may guide the course of treatment, they do not have the same legal standing as a living will or durable power of attorney for health care.

A non-legal document that may be used by a competent person along with a legal advance directive is the *values history form*, developed at the Center for Health Law and Ethics at the University of New Mexico. It consists of a series of questions dealing with such areas as one's attitudes toward health, toward one's life, toward independence and control, and toward illness, dying, and death; personal relationships; religious background and beliefs; and wishes concerning specific medical procedures. The values history form can substantially elaborate on the content of traditional advance directives and thus assist in medical treatment decision making. A sample values history form is included in Appendix 3 of this chapter.

The *Five Wishes* document, which is recognized as legally valid in some states, includes "not only the medical wishes but also the personal, emotional and spiritual wishes of seriously ill persons." (5) Its five sections cover "The Person I Want To Make Care Decisions for Me When I Can't," "The Kind of Medical Treatment I Want or Don't Want," "How Comfortable I Want To Be," "How I Want People to Treat Me," and "What I Want My Loved Ones to Know."

The concept of advance directives has now been extended to the realm of mental health. A "psychiatric advance directive" allows a mentally competent individual to tell a doctor, institution or judge what types of confinement and treatment he would or would not want and, if desired, to appoint an agent to make mental health care decisions if he himself becomes incapacitated to make them. (6)

FOR GROUP DISCUSSION

1. Consider the case of Ted Reed presented above. Given what you know about the nature of advance directives, do you think Ted should be hospitalized, given antibiotics, and placed on a ventilator? Why or why not?

2. To test your knowledge of advance directives, determine in each case whether advance directives are being correctly or incorrectly used.

   • Mrs. Charles, a resident of Crestridge Care Center, has terminal cancer. She suffers from some degree of mental confusion. Recently she has developed pneumonia. In view of her terminal illness, her physician thinks it appropriate to raise the question with her family whether antibiotics should be administered for the pneumonia. Mrs. Charles is a widow with five children, two daughters and three sons. She has executed a durable power of attorney for health care, naming her oldest daughter, Mary, as her proxy decision maker. The five children have a meeting and disagree about what should be done. Mary and her sister think that antibiotics should not be administered and that "nature should be allowed to take its course" for their mother. The three brothers, on the other hand, insist that the antibiotic treatment be administered. After the family conference the physician is told to administer the antibiotics because that is what the majority of Mrs. Charles's children want.

- Crestridge Care Center has a special unit for individuals suffering from various dementias. When a new resident is admitted, the person responsible for the resident is asked if he or she wishes to sign a living will for the individual being admitted.

- John Taylor, 78, is a resident of Crestridge Care Center who still takes walks around the neighborhood on his own. On one occasion he is hit by a car as he is crossing an intersection. When John is taken to the hospital emergency room, the ER staff pulls up his medical record on the hospital's computer system. The record shows that John has signed a living will. John is diagnosed as having a collapsed lung, a concussion, and a broken hip. Treatment is promptly begun, and five days later John is allowed to return to Crestridge Care Center to continue his recuperation.

- Roberta Thomas, 88, has been a resident of Crestridge Care Center for ten years. Recently, she suffered a serious stroke. She can no longer swallow and only has minimal awareness of what is going on. After talking with her physician, her family has begun their "death watch" around her bed. Upon entering the nursing home, Roberta had signed a living will. A decision is made not to hospitalize Roberta or to institute tube feedings to compensate for her inability to swallow, but to allow "nature to take its course" at this point.

- Richard Miller, 76, has been a resident in the dementia unit of Crestridge Care Center for ten years. When he retired at age 62, he had signed a durable power of attorney for health care in order to "prepare for the future," naming his oldest daughter as his proxy decision maker. Because of his advanced Alzheimer's disease, Richard has now "forgotten" how to eat. The issue has arisen of whether tube feeding should be started. Richard's wife and daughter have a conference with the facility's ethics committee to talk about this. After the ethics consult, Richard's wife tells the physician that she has decided that tube feeding should not be initiated for her husband.

- Leo Morris is a resident of Crestridge Care Center suffering from end-stage cancer. He is expected to live for a few more weeks, at the most. Although he is terminally ill, Leo remains lucid and alert. When Leo first learned three years ago that he had cancer, he signed a living will. Recently, Leo has begun to suffer from very low blood pressure, a problem he has had periodically throughout his life. Because of the fact that Leo has signed a living will, his physician does not even consider raising the issue of giving Leo medication for his dangerously low blood pressure.

- Leo Morris is a resident of Crestridge Care Center suffering from end-stage cancer. He is expected to live for a few more weeks, at the most. When Leo first learned three years ago that he had cancer, he signed a living will. Because he signed this document (which is in his medical record), his family assumes that no attempt will be made to resuscitate him at this point should he suffer a cardiac arrest. In their view, such an event would be a merciful way of ending his suffering.

- Alice Parker is another resident of Crestridge Care Center suffering from end-stage cancer. She is expected to live for a few more weeks, at the most. When she first learned three years ago that she had cancer, she signed a living will. At the present time Alice has started to experience severe pain. Her physician makes sure that she has adequate narcotic medication to keep her comfortable.

- Peter March, who is suffering from Alzheimer's disease, is a resident in the dementia unit of Crestridge Care Center. At the advice of the local Alzheimer's Association, he had executed a durable power of attorney for health care when he was still in the early stages of the disease and mentally competent to do so. In this document he named his son, Mark, as his proxy decision maker. Peter's physician discovers that Peter's kidneys are starting to fail and that he will soon need kidney dialysis. The physician consults Mark about whether this treatment should be undertaken. Mark decides that his father should not be started on dialysis. "Dad was a farmer who was always active physically and who liked to do things for himself," Mark states. "Alzheimer's disease has been very difficult for him to deal with," Mark reports, "and I'm sure he would never want to be hooked up to machines to keep him alive, especially when he can no longer understand what is really going on."

- Theresa McAlister is a resident of Crestridge Care Center. When she entered the facility, she executed a durable power of attorney for health care naming her daughter, Dolores, as her proxy decision maker. In this document she also specified that, if she ever reached the point of being confined to bed, she would want a Do-Not-Resuscitate order written. Theresa has recently suffered a stroke that has left her confined to her bed, in a semi-conscious state, and able to utter only a few disjointed words. Her physician indicates that her long-range prognosis is not good. A care conference is called with Dolores, and the issue is raised of obtaining a DNR order for Theresa. Dolores, however, objects, saying that her mother didn't necessarily know what is best to do medically. She says that it's too soon to give up hope of recovery for her mother.

3. In small groups, review the living will and durable power of attorney for health care documents for your state. (If you are connected with a long-term care facility, review as well the printed literature, videos, etc., used by the facility to explain these documents to residents.) Do you have any questions about the content of these documents? About how they should be filled out?

4. Individually, complete the values history form given in Appendix 3 of this chapter. Then discuss your responses in small groups. What have you learned through this exercise? Do you think that the values history form is a useful tool for medical treatment decision making and that its use should be encouraged? Why or why not?

NOTES

1. Commission on Legal Problems of the Elderly of the American Bar Association, "10 Legal Myths About Advance Directives." http://www.abanet.org/elderly/myths.html

2. Catholic Health Association of the United States, *The Patient Self-Determination Act* (St. Louis: Catholic Health Association, 1991).
3. Nancy M.P. King, *Making Sense of Advance Directives*, rev. ed. (Washington, DC: Georgetown University Press, 1996).
4. This case is adapted from "Mr. Woo" in Diane E. Hoffmann, Philip Boyle, & Steven A. Levenson, *Handbook for Nursing Home Ethics Committees* (Washington, D.C.: American Association of Homes and Services for the Aging, 1995).
5. *Five Wishes* can be obtained from Aging with Dignity, P.O. Box 1661, Tallahassee, Florida.
6. Judge David L. Bazelon Center for Mental Health Law, "Psychiatric Advance Directive," http://www.bazelon.org/advdir.html

ACKNOWLEDGMENTS

The sample living will form was developed by the Iowa State Bar Association, September, 1992.

The sample durable power of attorney for health care form was developed by the Medical-Moral Commission of the Archdiocese of Dubuque, Iowa, 1991.

The values history form is taken from the *Manual of Guidelines on Clinical-Ethical Issues* (St. Louis: Catholic Health Association, 1990), pp. 40-43.

FOR FURTHER STUDY

Additional Readings
- Eileen P. Flynn, *Your Living Will Why, When and How to Write One* (New York: Citadel Press, 1992). Also includes the durable power of attorney for health care.
- Lawrence P. Ulrich, *The Patient Self-Determination Act Meeting the Challenges in Patient Care* (Washington, DC: Georgetown University Press,1999).

Aids for implementing the use of advance directives within a facility or within the community
- *The Patient Self-Determination Act An Educational Resource* (St. Louis: Catholic Health Association of the United States, 1991). Although published by a religiously affiliated organization in health care, this three-ring binder of materials is largely nonsectarian. Sections include Education Module/Lesson Plan; Suggestions for Instructors; Documents for Developing Institutional Policy; Checklist for Administration; An Appendix containing the text of the Patient Self-Determination Act of 1990 with commentaries and information about the United States Supreme Court decision in the case of Nancy Cruzan; and a glossary and bibliography.
- *Respecting Your Choices*—Gundersen Lutheran Medical Center - La Crosse 1836-1910 South Ave. La Crosse, WI 54601 (Tel. 800-362-9567, ext. 4394. E-mail jabesl@lhl.gundluth.org) The *Respecting Your Choices* Program is a comprehensive approach to implementing an advance directives program in a health care setting and in the community. This program, which has been extremely successful in promoting the use of advance directives in the La Crosse, Wisconsin area, is described at http://www.gundluth.org/web/ptcare .

APPENDIX 1

Sample Living Will Form

DECLARATION RELATING TO THE USE OF LIFE-SUSTAINING PROCEDURES

DECLARATION

If I should have an incurable or irreversible condition that will result either in death within a relatively short period of time or a state of permanent unconsciousness from which, to a reasonable degree of medical certainty, there can be no recovery, it is my desire that my life not be prolonged by the administration of life-sustaining procedures. If I am unable to participate in my health care decisions, I direct my attending physician to withhold or withdraw life-sustaining procedures that merely prolong the dying process and are not necessary to my comfort or freedom from pain.

Signed this _____ day of _____ , 20 _____ .

_____

Signature of Person Making Declaration (Declarant)

_____

(Type or Print Name of Declarant)

_____

Street Address/City/State/Zip

This Declaration must be witnessed by two persons or be notarized.

STATE OF IOWA, _____ COUNTY, ss: _____

On this _____ day of _____ , A.D. 20 _____ , before me, the undersigned, a Notary Public in and for the State of Iowa, personally appeared _____ to me known to be the person named in and who executed the foregoing instrument as Declarant, and acknowledged that (he) (she) executed the same as (his) (her) voluntary act and deed.

_____ , Notary Public in and for said State.

By signing this form I declare that I signed this form in the presence of the other witness and the Declarant and I witnessed the signing by the Declarant or by another person acting on behalf of and at the Declarant's direction.

_____	_____
Signature of 1st Witness	Signature of 2nd Witness
_____	_____
(Type or Print Name of Witness)	(Type or Print Name of Witness)
_____	_____
Street Address	Street Address
_____	_____
City/State/Zip	City/State/Zip

127

APPENDIX 2

Sample Durable Power of Attorney for Health Care Form

CREATION OF POWER OF ATTORNEY FOR HEALTH CARE

I, the Principal, hereby designate

_____

First Name   Last Name

_____

(Type or Print) Street Address/City/State/Zip Code

as my attorney in fact (my agent) and give to my agent the power to make health care deci-sions for me. This power exists only when I am unable, in the judgment of my attending physician, to make those health care decisions. The attorney in fact must act consistently with my desires as stated in this document or otherwise made known.

Except as otherwise specified in this document, this document gives my agent the power, where otherwise consistent with the laws of the State of Iowa, to consent to my physician not giving health care or stopping health care which is necessary to keep me alive.

This document gives my agent power to make health care decisions on my behalf, including to consent, to refuse to consent, or to withdraw consent to any care, treatment, service, or procedure to maintain, diagnose, or treat a physical or mental condition. This power is sub-ject to any statement of my desires and any limitations included in this document. My agent has the right to examine my medical records and to consent to disclosure of such records.

SPECIFIC INSTRUCTIONS AND STATEMENT OF DESIRES

NOTE: The Principal does not have to give any specific instructions or statement of desires but may do so.

Insert here specific instructions or statement of desires of Principal (if any). Additional sheets may be attached.

DESIGNATION OF ALTERNATE HEALTH CARE AGENT

NOTE: The Principal may designate one or more alternates as attorney in fact but does not have to do so.

If the person designated above is unable to serve,

I designate

_____

First Name   Last Name

_____

(Type or Print) Street Address/City/State/Zip Code

to serve as my attorney in fact.

Signed this _____ day of _____, 20 _____

_____

Signature of Principal (Person Granting the Power of Attorney)

_____

Type or Print Name of Principal

_____

Street Address

_____

City/State/Zip Code

This Power of Attorney must either be witnessed by two persons OR notarized.

NOTARY PUBLIC

STATE OF IOWA, _____ COUNTY, ss: _____
On this _____ day of _____, A.D. 20 _____ , before me, the undersigned, a Notary Public in and for the State of Iowa, personally appeared _____ to me known to be the person named in and who executed the foregoing instrument as Declarant, and acknowledged that (he) (she) executed the same as (his) (her) voluntary act and deed.

_____ , Notary Public in and for said State.
By signing this form I declare that I signed this form in the presence of the other witness and the Declarant and I witnessed the signing by the Declarant or by another person acting on behalf of and at the Declarant's direction.

STATEMENT OF TWO WITNESSES

I know the Principal personally and I believe him or her to be of sound mind and at least 18 years of age. I believe that his or her signing of this power of attorney is voluntary. I am at least 18 years of age. I am not a health care provider for the Principal at this time.

_____   _____
Signature of 1st Witness   Signature of 2nd Witness

_____   _____
(Type or Print Name of Witness)   (Type or Print Name of Witness)

_____   _____
Street Address   Street Address

_____   _____
City/State/Zip   City/State/Zip

APPENDIX 3

Sample Values History

(Developed by the Center for Health Law and Ethics, University of New Mexico)

Your Thoughts about Specific Medical Questions

- Do you think it is a good idea to sign a legal document that says what medical treatments you do and do not want when you are dying?
- Do you think it is a good idea to sign a legal document that allows someone else to make health care decisions for you if you are unable to make these decisions yourself?
- Do you want to donate parts of your body to someone else at the time of your death?
- Do you think you would want to have any of the following medical treatments performed on you?
  - kidney dialysis
  - cardiopulmonary resuscitation
  - ventilator
  - artificial nutrition
  - artificial hydration

Questions about Your Life

A. *Your Health*
   - How do you feel about your current health?
   - If you have any medical problems, do they affect your ability to function? If yes, how?

B. *Your Doctors*
   - If you have a doctor, do you like him or her? Why?
   - Do you think your doctor should make the final decision about any medical treatments you might need?

C. *Your Independence*
   - Do you consider yourself an independent person?
   - Do you like to make our own decisions?
   - If you could not make your own decisions, would you be willing to let others make decisions for you?

D. *Your Personal Relationships*
   - Do you expect that your family and friends will support your decisions about any medical treatment you might need?
   - Have you made any arrangements for your family or friends to make medical decisions for you? If yes, who has agreed to make these decisions for you and in what circumstances?
   - If a member of your family were unable to make medical decisions, who should make the decisions for that person?

- Would you want to make medical decisions for members of your family or for your friends? If yes, in what circumstances?
- How do you feel about your relationships with your family?
- How do you feel about your relationships with your friends?

E. *Your Attitude Toward Life*
- What activities do you enjoy (e.g., hobbies, sports, watching TV, etc.)?
- Are you happy to be alive?
- Do you feel that your life is worth living?
- How satisfied are you with what you have done in your life?
- What makes you laugh? What makes you cry?
- What do you fear most? What frightens or upsets you?
- What goals do you have for the future?

F. *Your Attitude Toward Illness, Dying, and Death*
- Has anyone close to you died?
- What does death mean to you?
- What would you fear the most about a terminal illness?
- If you were to die tomorrow, are there any important unresolved matters you would want to settle today? If yes, what are they?
- Do you think you would like to plan your own funeral, or make decisions about your burial?

G. *Your Religious Beliefs*
- What are your beliefs about God or a higher power?
- Are you an active member of a church?
- Are prayer and worship important to you?
- How is death viewed in your religion?

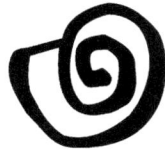

Chapter 13

Euthanasia and Assisted Suicide

Euthanasia and assisted suicide are both deliberate attempts to end a patient's life in order to end his or her suffering. These practices differ in the agent who introduces the immediate and direct cause of death. The act is called *euthanasia* when a person other than the patient directly does something to cause the patient's death. If a doctor injects a patient with an overdose of narcotic medication with the intent of bringing about the patient's death (perhaps in response to the patient's request), this is an act of euthanasia. *Assisted suicide* takes place when someone provides the patient with the means to take his or her own life but the patient is the one who directly initiates the action causing death. If a doctor deliberately prescribes medication so that a patient can take an overdose at home to cause his death, this is a case of assisted suicide. More specifically, this is a case of *physician assisted suicide (PAS)*.

Euthanasia is considered *voluntary* when it is undertaken at the request of or with the consent of the patient, *involuntary* when it is performed without the patient's consent. If a patient who is physically unable to take his own life asks a doctor to administer an overdose of a narcotic drug, this is an instance of voluntary euthanasia. If a physician administers an overdose of a narcotic drug to an elderly dementia patient solely at the request of the patient's children, this is a case of involuntary euthanasia.

Assisted suicide has practically become synonymous with the name of Dr. Jack Kevorkian, a retired pathologist in the State of Michigan. Some regard Dr. Kevorkian as a person on the fringes of medicine. But there are physicians in the mainstream of medical practice who favor (and practice) assisted suicide and euthanasia. Quite a stir was caused by the appearance of an article, "It's Over, Debbie," in the prestigious *Journal of the American Medical Association*. It was written by a medical resident (whose name was withheld) who gave a twenty-year-old woman dying of ovarian cancer a lethal injection of morphine. (1)

The possibility of assisted suicide or euthanasia is considered in three different types of situations: (a) the patient is in the final stages of the dying process; (b) the patient has a progressively debilitating disease; and (c) the patient has a terminal condition or a severely debilitating disease and is in severe pain.

This chapter covers:
- *arguments given in favor of euthanasia and assisted suicide;*
- *objections raised against euthanasia and assisted suicide;*
- *the legal status of these practices;*

- *whether there is a difference between forgoing life-sustaining treatments and the practices of euthanasia and assisted suicide;*
- *the movement toward better care of the dying as an alternative to euthanasia and assisted suicide.*

CASE STUDIES

Mrs. Janet Redmond, 92, has been a resident of the Carlisle Nursing Home for twelve years. She is quite frail and suffers from very low blood pressure which requires medication. To make things worse, she has had pneumonia three times in the last four months.

One evening Janet suffers a mild stroke. Her family, two sons and a daughter, are called to the nursing home. The eldest son, Richard, is designated as proxy decision maker in his mother's durable power of attorney for health care. After conferring with his brother and sister, Richard agrees to have a feeding tube placed since his mother is only semiconscious and unable to swallow.

After a few days Janet seems to begin recovering from the stroke. She recognizes family members who come to visit her. Her children are hopeful that she will come out of this, just as she recovered from the three bouts of pneumonia when no one expected her to do so.

However, a week later Janet suffers another and more serious stroke. Her physician, Dr. Hart, tells the family that it is only a matter of time before Janet dies. Janet's children begin the "death watch" around her bed. At this point Janet seems to have no awareness of her environment and does not respond to the words or loving touches of her family. She is quite agitated, continually tossing and turning in bed and pulling at the feeding tube.

At the suggestion of Dr. Hart, Richard agrees to withdrawal of the feeding tube and to stopping his mother's blood pressure medication. Stopping treatments and allowing death to come, he believes, would be a merciful end to his mother's suffering.

However, Janet lingers on for another week. Her daughter, Carolyn, herself a nurse, approaches Dr. Hart about giving her mother a muscle-relaxing injection to paralyze her lungs. Carolyn tells Dr. Hart that she loves her mother too much to allow her to continue to suffer in this way. Somewhat to her surprise, Dr. Hart agrees to Carolyn's request.

At ten o'clock that evening, Dr. Hart goes to the nursing home. Dr. Hart tells the nursing staff on duty that he wants to check on his long-time patient, Janet Redmond, but has been so busy that day that he couldn't come until now. He surreptitiously administers the injection, then leaves. Half an hour later, a nurse on duty finds Janet Redmond dead.

The nursing staff is surprised about Janet's death. A nurse who had checked on her just an hour before had not noticed any sudden deterioration in her condition. And it's most unusual—and downright suspicious—for a physician to visit a nursing home at that time of night. The nursing staff wonders if they should inform the family about these circumstances, or simply tell them that their mother has died. Indeed, they wonder if they should push for an investigation into the cause of Janet's death.

*　　*　　*

At age 70, Dr. Ralph Cox retires from family practice in a rural midwestern community. The first two years of his retirement are good ones, giving him the opportunity to spend time with his six grandchildren. But then his wife, Ruth, begins to notice behavioral changes in him. After he "got lost" driving home one afternoon, they both agree that he should be checked out medically. It is learned that Dr. Cox is in the very early stages of Alzheimer's disease.

To make matters worse, Ruth dies unexpectedly a year later. At this point, Ralph decides to enter Glenview Village, a multi-level facility, in order to "prepare for the future." Initially, Ralph resides in an assisted living apartment, but, being a physician, he knows what is to come as the disease progresses. And, apart from his Alzheimer's disease, his eyesight is beginning to fail and he is starting to have difficulty walking because of arthritis.

Ralph has three children, Monica, Mark, and Amy. Mark and Amy live out of state, so the main caregiving responsibilities fall on Ralph's oldest daughter Monica who lives in a nearby city. Monica drives to Glenview Village daily to see her father, usually spending two or three hours with him and taking care of needs around the apartment. Monica never complains, but Ralph worries that she is taking too much time away from her own husband and children in order to care for him. Ralph also worries about the high cost of his present and future care. He knows that people with Alzheimer's disease can still live for a long time, and, as a rural physician, his retirement "nest egg" really isn't all that much. He doesn't want his children to have to assume the cost of his care, especially with children of their own to educate.

Ralph dearly loves his six grandchildren, and much prizes the time he has spent with them since his retirement. He wants them to have good memories of their grandfather. He dreads the idea that they will eventually see him in a demented, debilitated state.

During the winter, Ralph develops pneumonia. He refuses to take the antibiotics prescribed for him. Because of his arthritis, he has to use a cane when walking. He can tell that he is getting more forgetful and must constantly write things down on paper for himself.

One afternoon Ralph begs Monica to contact the Hemlock Society to "help him end it all." Monica sympathizes with her father's deteriorating condition, but vigorously disagrees with his request. Monica is so upset by her father's request for assisted suicide that she contacts the social worker at Glenview Village, Marvin Dalton. Monica and Marvin had been classmates in high school, so she feels free to share her distress with him. Marvin suggests that Monica contact Ralph's pastor to help the whole family work through this.

The Defense of Euthanasia and Assisted Suicide

What are the arguments that might be offered in support of acts of euthanasia and assisted suicide? How do people try to justify it?

First and most fundamentally, these practices are defended as being acts of compassion in relieving suffering. In the first case scenario, Janet Redmond is in the final stages of the dying process. She is unaware of her environment and unresponsive to her family. She is obviously uncomfortable, tossing and turning in bed. Life-sustaining treatments (the feeding tube and blood pressure medications) have been withdrawn, but she lingers on. Why make her suffer any longer? Why not compassionately end her suffering now, as Dr. Hart in fact did? After all, it is accepted practice to put animals out of their misery. Should we not be at least as kind to human beings?

Another argument offered in favor of euthanasia and assisted suicide is that these practices promote death with dignity. People today may not fear death so much as they fear the dying process, which brings about debilitation and dependency. With euthanasia and assisted suicide, a patient can end his life when he is still "himself," and be remembered that way by his loved ones. This argument applies to the case of Ralph Cox, who does not want his grandchildren to have as their last memories of him pictures of a debilitated, demented Alzheimer's patient.

A value much emphasized in contemporary health care ethics is patient autonomy. Some see deciding on the time of one's death as the ultimate exercise of self-determination. According to this line of argument, if Ralph Cox is still judged mentally competent and wants to end his life, it is his right to do so.

It is generally recognized that taking human life can sometimes be legitimate. Examples might be self-defense, the killing that takes place during a war and, some would add, capital punishment. It might be argued that this list should be expanded to include euthanasia and assisted suicide for the terminally ill and for those suffering from irreversible, progressively debilitating diseases (like multiple sclerosis). Indeed, there are some instances in which people do something to bring about their own deaths that we consider morally commendable. Consider the classic case of someone voluntarily jumping out of an overcrowded lifeboat so that others can survive, or the case of a soldier falling on a grenade to save his buddies, or the Buddhist monks who burned themselves to death in protest over the Viet Nam war.

Ralph Cox fears the mounting bills for his care and believes he is a burden to his oldest daughter. If a patient chooses to take his own life in order to relieve his family of the financial burdens and the strains of caregiving, isn't this a commendable thing to do?

Objections to Euthanasia and Assisted Suicide

Arguments against euthanasia and assisted suicide have been put forward on both religious and non-religious grounds. Since American society is pluralistic with many differing views on religion, we will begin by considering the non-religious arguments.

First of all, medical diagnoses and prognoses can be mistaken. We all know of people who were told they had a short life expectancy because of a disease, and then unexpectedly recovered or substantially outlived the projections for "how much time they had left." Since medical diagnoses and prognoses are not 100 percent sure, the concern is that, if assisted suicide and euthanasia are allowed, some people may end their lives needlessly or prematurely. (2) For example, in the case of Janet Redmond, her physician is of the opinion that she will not survive. But she might unexpectedly rally and survive for some time. After all, she has had her ups and downs with three bouts of pneumonia and recovered when no one expected her to do so.

Second, there is always the possibility of a breakthrough occurring in medical research, making a treatment available that would improve the condition of a patient with a particular disease. This consideration would apply, for example, to the case of Ralph Cox with Alzheimer's disease. Euthanasia and assisted suicide close off this option. (2)

Ralph Cox is coping with progressively declining health. In addition to the progress of Alzheimer's disease, his eyesight is beginning to fail and he has to use a cane to walk because of arthritis. He has suffered a bout of pneumonia. Such debilitating illnesses can cause a patient to become depressed. Even apart from clinical depression, serious illness can distort a patient's judgment:

> Anyone who has been severely ill knows how distorted his judgment became during the worst moments of the illness. Pain and the toxic effect of disease, or the violent reaction to certain surgical procedures may change our capacity for rational and courageous thought. (3)

While it may be true that "some euthanasia candidates will have their lucid moments," yet "how they are to be distinguished from fellow-sufferers who do not, or how these instances are to be distinguished from others when the patient is exercising an irrational judgment, is not an easy matter." (3) Moreover, it is not unusual for a patient to undergo mood changes during the course of a day so that he may want euthanasia or assisted suicide "during the morning depression" but "later in the day he will think quite differently, or will have forgotten all about it." (3) All these psychological factors can skew a patient's judgment in requesting an end to his life so that the request does not represent his true, rational, underlying desires.

There is also a concern that patients who are difficult or expensive to take care of may feel pressured by other people into opting for euthanasia or assisted suicide when they really do not want this:

Will we not sweep up, in the process, some who are not really tired of life, but think others are tired of them; some who do not really want to die, but who feel they should not live on, because to do so when there looms the legal alternative of euthanasia is to do a selfish or cowardly act? Will not some feel an obligation to have themselves "eliminated" in order that funds allocated for their terminal care might be better used by their families or, financial worries aside, in order to relieve their families of the emotional strain involved? (3)

Note that, in the second case scenario, Ralph Cox "worries about the high cost of his present and future care" and about the possibility of his children having to assume the cost of his care, and is concerned about his daughter Monica "taking too much time away from her own husband and children in order to care for him."

Further, there is fear that a slippery slope effect will occur. In other words, there is fear that if we allow euthanasia and assisted suicide in some cases, the practice will expand to include other cases in which it really is not justifiable. For example, we might start out with voluntary euthanasia and assisted suicide, wherein life is ended at the request of the patient. But this might expand to cases of involuntary euthanasia in which someone other than the patient decides that a patient's life is to be ended. (Just consider the first case scenario in which Dr. Hart and Janet Redmond's daughter Carolyn are the ones who decide that Janet's life is to be ended by the injection of a muscle-relaxing drug which paralyzes the lungs.) Or again, we might start out with allowing euthanasia and assisted suicide for those who are terminally ill and find it expanding to those whose conditions are not life threatening and may be treatable. This phenomenon has already occurred in the practice of Dr. Jack Kevorkian. The thirty-fifth person he helped commit suicide was Judith Curren, a woman suffering from chronic fatigue syndrome, a weight problem, and depression. (4)

Finally, euthanasia and assisted suicide must be considered from the perspective of health care professionals and services. The American Medical Association has commented that "physician assisted suicide is fundamentally incompatible with the physician's role as healer." (5) And it is argued that "physician-assisted suicide could...undermine the trust that is essential to the doctor-patient relationship by blurring the time-honored line between healing and harming." (5)

At present, health care workers are dedicated to saving lives, even to the point of taking a patient's death as a personal failure. (2) If euthanasia and assisted suicide were accepted practices, "doctors and nurses might not try hard enough to save the patient" in cases of severe illness and "decide that the patient would simply be 'better off dead.'" (2) Indeed, "this attitude could then carry over to their dealings with patients less seriously ill" so that the "result would be an overall decline in the quality of medical care." (2)

Religious Opposition to Euthanasia and Assisted Suicide

In the second case scenario Ralph Cox's daughter Monica is advised to contact their pastor to help them work through Ralph's request for assisted suicide. For the most part, religious denominations have traditionally opposed the practices of euthanasia and assisted suicide. (6) Coming from a religious perspective, what might the pastor say?

First of all, the pastor might point out that all life is sacred and that taking life is prohibited in the Ten Commandments. (2) Further, the pastor might tell Ralph that life is a gift from God and that we are merely stewards, not owners, of our lives. It is not our prerogative to dispose of our lives as we wish; rather, taking life is the prerogative of God. (2) This mentality is diametrically opposed to the argument from autonomy given in support of euthanasia and assisted suicide.

Ralph's pastor might also remind him that, from a religious perspective, suffering is of value. (7) As this idea has been articulated in a Christian context:

> ...it is true that life often presents us with painful circumstances, and we may be inclined to consider suicide as a way of avoiding this suffering. But for the true Christian, suffering is to be *welcomed*, not avoided. For the true Christian, mere happiness is not the goal of life; rather, the true Christian seeks the attainment of blessedness, moral elevation, and eternal life. But the way to salvation is *through* suffering: one must therefore submit oneself willingly to suffering... To commit suicide in order to avoid suffering would be to fail to see it as the means to grace. (7)

In particular, at least some suffering is claimed to have a "morally educative character" in that it engenders virtuous traits such as depth of sympathy, love, flexibility, humility, and self-reliance. (7)

Natural law ethics is associated with the Roman Catholic tradition. Basically, this theory maintains that an action that is in accord with what is natural is right, but an action that goes against what is natural is wrong. (See the Appendix on Ethical Theory.) Euthanasia and assisted suicide are seen as going against the natural human inclination for self-preservation, and therefore are judged morally wrong:

> ...Every human being has a natural inclination to continue living. Our reflexes and responses fit us to fight against attackers, flee wild animals, and dodge out of the way of trucks. In our daily lives we exercise the caution and care necessary to protect ourselves. Our bodies are similarly structured for survival right down to the molecular level. When we are cut, our capillaries seal shut, our blood clots, and fibrin is produced to start the process of healing the wound. When we are invaded by bacteria, antibodies are produced to fight against the alien organisms, and their remains are swept out of the body by special cells designed for clean-up work...

It is enough, I believe, to recognize that the organization of the human body and our patterns of behavioral responses make the continuation of life a natural goal. By reason alone, then, we can recognize that euthanasia sets us against our own nature. (2)

Opposition to euthanasia and assisted suicide is by no means limited to the Catholic religious tradition. Robert Wennberg, a philosophy professor and Presbyterian minister, raises concerns about these practices from the perspective of their impact on other people:

...Christian believers contemplating the possibility of surcease suicide, fraught with moral danger as it is, must also take into account the impact of such an action upon the community of faith of which they are a part and which they hold dear, and upon the larger uncommitted community of which they are also a part. For such an act of life termination may be perceived as a shocking rejection of God's rightful sovereignty over life and death, as a repudiation of God as a sufficient source of strength in time of trouble, as a raging against divinely appointed suffering, and, finally, as an act of total spiritual despair. (8)

In sum, Wennberg proposes that "suicide is a questionable vehicle for making a Christian statement about the meaning of life by the manner of one's death, in part because of how that death will be understood and possibly misunderstood by others." (8)

The Legal Debate

The practice of assisted suicide has provoked legal activity at both state and national levels. Dr. Jack Kevorkian has been brought to trial more than once for his activities in the State of Michigan, and in March 1999, he was convicted of second-degree murder for giving a fatal injection to a man with a terminal illness. Several states have had ballot initiatives to legalize physician assisted suicide (PAS). While some have failed, a ballot initiative was passed by a narrow margin in Oregon in 1994 and ratified in a general election in 1997. (9)

In June 1997, the U.S. Supreme Court rendered a judgment in two cases concerning assisted suicide, *Washington v. Glucksberg* and *Vacco v. Quill*. The Court "denied that assistance by physicians in suicide is a constitutionally protected right of terminally ill persons and their physicians." (9) At the same time, the Court did not completely rule out assisted suicide, but put this question in the hands of the states. Six Justices stated in their opinions that state legislatures remain the appropriate forum in which decriminalizing (and thus permitting) some kind of carefully controlled physician assistance in dying can be examined and, perhaps, experiments with it undertaken. (9)

The two cases taken to the Supreme Court explicitly raised question about a *distinction* which has been commonly made and used in health care. The legitimacy of forgoing (that is, withholding or withdrawing) life-sustaining treatments has long been recognized. At the same time, forgoing life-sustaining treatments has been seen as much different from the (impermissible) practices of euthanasia and assisted suicide. But is there really a difference between, for example, taking someone off a ventilator so that death can take place and providing a patient with an overdose of medication to bring on death? Are not both actions taken to *hasten death*? So shouldn't assisted suicide be recognized and allowed as just another form of an already accepted practice? (10)

In the decision in *Vacco v. Quill* Chief Justice Rehnquist took the significant step of reaffirming the traditional distinction:

> Unlike the court of appeals, we think the distinction between assisting suicide and withdrawing life-sustaining treatment, a distinction widely recognized and endorsed in the medical profession and in our legal traditions, is both important and logical; it is certainly rational. (11)

But exactly what is the difference between "killing" and "letting die"? It is often explained in terms of the cause of death:

> ...as a reality of nature, killing and letting die are causally different. "Letting die" is only physically possible if there is some underlying disease that will serve as the cause of death. Put me on a ventilator now, when I am in good health, and nothing whatever will happen if it is turned off. I cannot be "allowed to die" by having a ventilator turned off if I have healthy lungs. It is wholly different, however, if a doctor gives me a muscle-relaxing injection that will paralyze my lungs. Healthy or not, those lungs will cease to function and I will die. This is what it means to "kill" someone as distinguished from "letting" someone die. Put more formally, there must be an underlying fatal pathology if allowing to die is even possible. Killing, by contrast, provides its own fatal pathology. Nothing but the action of the doctor giving the lethal injection is necessary to bring about death. (12)

When a life-sustaining treatment is forgone, there is an underlying disease that is allowed to take its course and that directly causes death. A natural disease process brings about death. In euthanasia or assisted suicide, on the other hand, an intentional human action is the direct and immediate cause of death.

Consider the death of Janet Redmond in the first case scenario. Suppose she had died after the feeding tube was removed and her blood pressure medication stopped. Her death would have been due to her stroke and to her cardiovascular problems. But her death did not happen this way. The direct and immediate cause of her death was the muscle-relaxing drug injected by Dr. Hart, which paralyzed her lungs. Dr. Hart engaged in an act of euthanasia.

The Oregon Experiment

The 1997 U.S. Supreme Court decision on assisted suicide permits states to conduct experiments with this practice. Oregon's Death with Dignity Act allows a patient to request a prescription for lethal medication from a licensed Oregon physician. To make this request, an individual must be 18 years of age or older, a resident of Oregon, "capable" (that is, able to make and communicate health care decisions), and diagnosed with a terminal illness that will lead to death within six months. (13) The following steps must be taken to receive a prescription for lethal medication:

- The patient must make two oral requests to his or her physician, separated by at least 15 days.

- The patient must provide a written request to his or her physician, signed in the presence of two witnesses.

- The patient's diagnosis and prognosis must be confirmed by the prescribing physician and by a consulting physician.

- The prescribing physician and a consulting physician must determine whether the patient is "capable."

- The patient must be referred for a psychological examination if either physician believes that the patient's judgment is impaired by a psychiatric or psychological disorder.

- The prescribing physician must inform the patient of feasible alternatives to assisted suicide including comfort care, hospice care, and pain control.

- The prescribing physician must request, but may not require, the patient to notify his or her next-of-kin of the prescription request. (13)

According to the provisions of the Oregon law, physicians must report to the state all prescriptions for lethal medications, and pharmacists must be informed of the prescribed medication's ultimate use. (13) Particular physicians and healthcare systems are not mandated to participate in the practice of physician assisted suicide (13), and thus may opt out of it for reasons of conscience.

Since the Oregon law went into effect, the following statistics have been compiled on the use of physician assisted suicide (PAS):

> In 2001, a total of 44 prescriptions of lethal doses of medication were written by 33 physicians. By comparison, 39 prescriptions were written in 2000, 33 in 1999 and 24 in 1998. Nineteen of the fourth-year prescription recipients died after ingesting the medication; 14 died from their underlying disease and 11 were alive on December 31, 2001. In addition, two patients who received prescriptions during 2000 died in 2001 after ingesting their medication for a total of 21 PAS deaths during 2001. This compares to 27 PAS deaths in 2000, 27 in 1999, and 16 in 1998. (13)

In the year 2001, one half of the patients using the prescribed lethal medication became unconscious within three minutes after ingesting it and died within 25 minutes. One patient vomited after ingesting the medication and died 25 hours later; another patient lived for 37 hours after ingestion. Neither of these patients, however, regained consciousness, nor were emergency medical services called. (13)

In comparison with residents of Oregon dying from similar underlying causes, the 21 patients who used PAS during 2001 were slightly more likely to be women, more likely to have graduated from college, and more likely to be divorced. Cancer was the predominant underlying illness. The most commonly mentioned end-of-life concerns voiced by these individuals were a loss of autonomy, a decreasing ability to participate in activities that made life enjoyable, and losing control of bodily functions. (13)

Towards Better Care of the Dying

The societal movement towards euthanasia and assisted suicide did not arise in a vacuum. Opponents of these practices see this movement as resulting from a failure to provide good care for the dying:

> Many who care for the dying tell us that people are generally not afraid to die. They fear, rather, the process of dying, especially the dependency, helplessness, and pain that so often accompany terminal illness...

> One of the major arguments of euthanasia advocates is that for some people dying is too painful to endure and so bringing about death by lethal injection or assisted suicide is the only merciful way to end the pain and suffering. (14)

Thus, some opponents of euthanasia and assisted suicide are campaigning for better palliative care for the dying. (9) Recognizing that a cure cannot be achieved, this is medical care aimed at relieving pain and other distressing symptoms of the dying process. (See the chapter "Pain Management.") Hospice programs are a prime example of palliative care. As one proponent of palliative care states it, "...people involved in health care have now what may be a brief window of opportunity to increase their efforts to improve and refine palliative medicine and hospice practice so that fewer and fewer persons imagine that PAD [physician-assisted dying] is their only hope, as they live in fear of unrelieved suffering and indignity in their dying as a consequence of medical neglect." (9)

The suffering that accompanies the dying process goes beyond physical pain. Providing emotional and psychological support for those who are ill is likewise advocated as part of good care of the dying. As stated in one document opposing euthanasia:

> The pleas of gravely ill people who sometimes ask for death are not to be understood as implying a true desire for euthanasia; in fact it is almost always a case of an anguished plea for help and love. What a sick person needs, besides medical care, is love, the human and supernatural warmth with which the sick person can and ought to be surrounded by all those close to him or her, parents and children, doctors and nurses. (15)

> As for those who work in the medical profession, they ought to neglect no means of making all their skill available to the sick and the dying; but they should also remember how much more necessary it is to provide them with the comfort of boundless kindness and heartfelt charity. (15)

Advancing the cause of palliative care is one area in which proponents and opponents of euthanasia and assisted suicide may find some common ground. For even some who believe euthanasia and assisted suicide are morally permissible in some cases still advocate trying palliative care as the first course of action:

> The new Quill plan proposes to use palliative care experts to review all requests for assisted suicide or euthanasia. The specialist in comfort care would talk with the patient and primary physician, and review the medical records and treatments that have already been used. ...if the palliative care doctor finds that the patient's request for euthanasia comes from inadequate treatment of his symptoms, wrote Quill and his colleagues, "The process of consultation might lead to improved pain management or the use of other means of comfort care." In any case, a patient who had not yet received adequate comfort care would be offered better treatment of symptoms, not death. (16)

FOR GROUP DISCUSSION

1. In the first case scenario the nursing staff is concerned about the cause of Janet Redmond's death and about the actions of Dr. Hart. Let's suppose they decide to inform Mrs. Redmond's family about the circumstances surrounding their mother's death, and to confront Dr. Hart directly about their concerns.

   - Role play a meeting called to discuss this incident. Those involved should include Dr. Hart, Janet's three children (Richard, Carolyn, and another son), several members of the nursing staff on duty at the time, and the nursing home's administrator.

   - After listening to this meeting and thinking critically about the material presented in this chapter, do you think it was morally permissible for Dr. Hart to bring about Janet Redmond's death?

2. Consider again the case of Janet Redmond. If she had died after removal of the feeding tube and cessation of the blood pressure medication, we would be dealing with a case of forgoing a life-sustaining treatment, a practice that is accepted. As things stand, we are dealing with a case of involuntary euthanasia in that her death was immediately caused by an injection of a muscle-relaxing drug that paralyzed her lungs and was decided upon by her daughter and her physician. Do you personally feel there is a difference between forgoing a life-sustaining treatment and euthanasia/assisted suicide? Explain your response.

3. Suppose you are involved in caring for a terminally ill patient who, like Ralph Cox, pleads with you to "help me die." How would you react? What would you say to this patient?

4. If you are connected with a religious-sponsored facility, research that denomination's views on euthanasia and assisted suicide. A good place to begin your research is Laurence J. O'Connell's *Active Euthanasia, Religion, and the Public Debate* published by the Park Ridge Center in Chicago in 1991. Discuss the denomination's position and the reasons behind it.

5. The United States Supreme Court has left it to individual states to decide whether to allow and experiment with assisted suicide. Have any initiatives been undertaken in your state to legalize assisted suicide? What conditions are being proposed to govern the practice of assisted suicide? What is your own response to this (proposed) legislation?

6. Oregon's Death with Dignity Act requires the physician prescribing the lethal medication to inform the patient of feasible alternatives to assisted suicide including comfort care, hospice care, and pain control. Is this requirement in Oregon law satisfactory? In other words, do you think that most physicians have sufficient training in palliative care to be able to present to terminally ill patients feasible alternatives to assisted suicide? Or should there be a requirement that a physician with special training in palliative care review all requests for assisted suicide? (17)

7. In the midst of the debate about physician assisted suicide, another course of action being discussed is *patient refusal of nutrition and hydration*. PRNH refers to the conscious refusal of nutrition and hydration on the part of a terminally ill patient even though the patient may be able to take food orally. The patient's intent is to hasten death, with death usually occurring within one to two weeks. PRNH is advocated on the grounds that it represents a reasonably comfortable way of dying, that it is a simpler procedure in avoiding any legal requirements for qualifying for physician assisted suicide (such as those set by the state of Oregon), and that it avoids complicity on the part of health care providers in the death of the patient. (18)

   • In your view, does PRNH qualify as "suicide"? Is it any different than a refusal of artificial nutrition and hydration on the part of a terminally ill person?

   • In long-term care it is not unusual for a resident to have no desire for food and to express no hunger and then to die shortly thereafter. This reaction is interpreted as a natural shutting down of the body in the dying process. Is this situation different than PRNH? If so, how can the two cases be differentiated?

   • Would you feel comfortable raising the option of PRNH with a resident who is dying? Do you personally think that PRNH is an ethically permissible practice?

NOTES

1. Anonymous, "It's Over, Debbie," *Journal of the American Medical Association* 259/2 (Jan. 8, 1988): 272.
2. J. Gay-Williams, "The Wrongfulness of Euthanasia" in Ronald Munson (ed.), *Intervention and Reflection Basic Issues in Medical Ethics*, 5th ed. (Belmont, CA:Wadsworth, 1996).
3. Yale Kamisar, "From Euthanasia Legislation: Some Non-Religious Objections" in A.B. Downing (ed.), *Euthanasia and the Right to Die* (New York: Humanities Press, 1970).

4. Chicago Tribune, "Kevorkian Steps Over a Fine Line" reprinted in the (Dubuque) *Telegraph-Herald*, August 23, 1996.

5. Chief Justice Rehnquist, From the Decision in *Washington v. Glucksberg*, *New York Times*, June 27, 1997.

6. Laurence J. O'Connell, *Active Euthanasia, Religion, and the Public Debate* (Chicago: The Park Ridge Center, 1991).

7. Margaret Pabst Battin, *Ethical Issues in Suicide* (Englewood Cliffs, NJ: Prentice-Hall, 1982).

8. Robert N. Wennberg, *Terminal Choices Euthanasia, Suicide, and the Right to Die* (Grand Rapids, MI: William B. Eerdmans, 1989), p. 101.

9. James F. Bresnahan, "Palliative Care or Assisted Suicide?" *America* (March 14, 1998): 16-21.

10. James F. Bresnahan, "Killing vs. Letting Die A Moral Distinction Before the Courts," *America* (Feb. 1, 1997): 8-16.

11. Chief Justice Rehnquist, From the Decision in *Vacco v. Quill*, *New York Times*, June 27, 1997.

12. Daniel Callahan, *The Troubled Dream of Life In Search of a Peaceful Death* (New York: Simon & Schuster, 1993).

13. Oregon Public Health Services, Center for Health Statistics and Vital Records, *Oregon's Death with Dignity Act Annual Report 2001*; see http://www.ohd.hr.state.or.us/chs/pas

14. Catholic Health Association of the United States, *Care of the Dying A Catholic Perspective* (St. Louis: Catholic Health Association of the United States, 1993).

15. Vatican Congregation for the Doctrine of the Faith, *Declaration on Euthanasia* (Washington, DC: United States Catholic Conference, 1980).

16. Lonny Shavelson, *A Chosen Death The Dying Confront Assisted Suicide* (New York: Simon & Schuster, 1995). The reference is to Dr. Timothy Quill.

17. Kathleen Foley and Herbert Hendin, "The Oregon Report: Don't Ask, Don't Tell," *Hastings Center Report* (May-June 1999), available at http://www.ortl.org/suicide/oregon_report.html

18. Ira R. Byock, "Patient Refusal of Nutrition and Hydration: Walking the Ever-Finer Line," *American Journal of Hospice & Palliative Care* (March/April 1995): 8-13, available at http://www.dyingwell.com/prnh.htm

FOR FURTHER STUDY

• Lonny Shavelson, *A Chosen Death The Dying Confront Assisted Suicide* (New York: Simon & Schuster, 1995). Shavelson is a writer, photojournalist, and emergency room physician who presents the stories of five terminally ill patients who wrestle with the decision of whether to end their lives.

• Ron Dzwonkowski (ed.), *The Suicide Machine: Understanding Jack Kevorkian, the People Who Came to Him, and the Issue of Assisted Suicide* (Detroit, MI: Detroit Free Press, 1997).

• Task Force to Improve the Care of Terminally Ill Oregonians, *The Oregon Death with Dignity Act A Guidebook for Healthcare Providers* (Portland, OR: OHSU Center for Ethics in Health Care).

- National Hospice Organization Ethics Committee (ed.), *Proactive Responses to the Assisted Suicide Euthanasia Debate* (National Hospice Organization, 1996).

- Timothy E. Quill, *Death and Dignity: Making Choices and Taking Charge* (NY: W.W. Norton, 1994). Dr. Quill is a physician in the mainstream of medical practice who advocates and has practiced assisted suicide.

- Herbert Hendin, *Seduced by Death: Doctors, Patients, and Assisted Suicide*, rev. ed. (NY: W.W. Norton, 1998). Written by a psychiatrist, this book argues against legalized assisted suicide. The previous edition was cited by the U.S. Supreme Court in its 1997 decision on physician assisted suicide.

- Herbert Hendin and Kathleen M. Foley (eds.), *Case against Assisted Suicide: For the Right to End-of-Life Care* (Baltimore: Johns Hopkins University Press, 2002).

- Ronald P. Hamel and Edwin R. DuBose (eds.), *Must We Suffer Our Way to Death? Cultural and Theological Perspectives on Death by Choice* (Dallas: Southern Methodist University Press, 1996).

- Edwin R. DuBose, *Physician Assisted Suicide: Religious and Public Policy Implications* (Chicago: Park Ridge Center, 2001).

- Episcopal Committee on Medical Ethics, *Assisted Suicide and Euthanasia: Christian Moral Perspectives* (Morehouse Publishing, 1997). This book looks at the full range of arguments on assisted suicide and euthanasia that can be given from within the Christian tradition.

Part Three

Issues of Professionalism

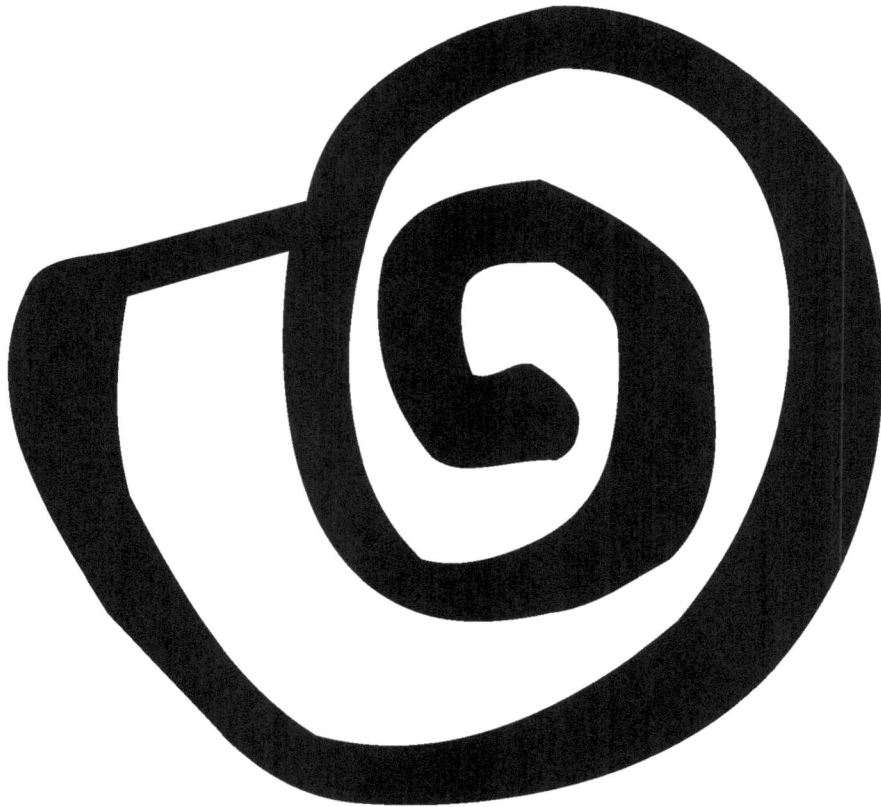

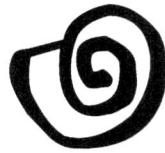

Chapter 14

Confidentiality

Leaks of supposedly confidential or privileged information to the media have become commonplace in American society. This attitude may make it harder to appreciate why confidentiality is emphasized and expected in health care. Yet confidentiality goes back to the Hippocratic oath: "Whatever I see or hear, professionally or privately, which ought not be divulged, I will keep secret and tell no one." (1)

This chapter covers:
- *the reasons why confidentiality is an important value in health care;*
- *the ethical principle governing confidentiality;*
- *when it is ethically legitimate to break confidentiality;*
- *the challenge of preserving confidentiality in computerized health information;*
- *HIPAA regulations regarding health care information.*

CASE STUDIES

Jerry Miller works as a certified nursing assistant (CNA) at St. Francis Home, a multi-level care facility. While he is shopping in the grocery store one evening, an elderly neighbor, Irma Todd, stops to talk with him. Irma is a regular at the community's senior center, and she knows that one of her card partners, Larry Steffen, has recently been admitted to St. Francis Home for a period of recuperation after hip replacement surgery. She asks Jerry how Larry is doing.

Without thinking, Jerry gives Irma a fairly detailed report on Larry's condition and the progress he is making towards recovery. After all, she seems as concerned about him as if he were her own husband!

* * *

Dolores Porter, the Director of Nursing (DON) at St. Francis Home, has requested a special meeting of the facility's ethics committee. She wants to discuss a problem that has arisen with a widowed male resident, 75, who is in the assisted living apartments.

Dolores tells the ethics committee that a housekeeper discovered a bottle of a drug prescribed to enhance sexual potency in this man's apartment. This is a matter of concern to her because other sections of St. Francis Home have female residents suffering from mild to moderate dementia who sometimes wander, and hard as staff may try, they can't watch these women every single minute of the day. Although St. Francis Home has three different buildings for different levels of care, there are walkways connecting the buildings. Dolores is afraid that the male resident in question may entice these women into his apartment and, given their diminished mental capacities, easily entrap them into having sex with him.

Dolores informs the ethics committee that she has tried speaking with this resident on several occasions about his possession and use of the drug, but he absolutely refuses to discuss the matter. She also informs the ethics committee that she called the physician who prescribed the drug to explain her concerns, but that she got nowhere with this physician. The doctor told her that the man in question is still fully competent mentally, and that such a prescription is a matter solely between a doctor and his patient.

Dolores wonders if she should contact this man's two children to tell them about the drug their father has obtained and alert them to the potential problems with their father and the safety of other residents. She also hopes that they would be willing to try to persuade their father to relinquish the drug. However, contacting the children would involve divulging medical information without this man's consent. It is for this reason that Dolores has come to seek the advice of the ethics committee.

Recognizing Issues of Confidentiality

These cases raise the ethical issue of confidentiality several times. First, there is the CNA, Jerry, who gives out medical information about a nursing home resident in casual conversation with a concerned neighbor. This seems harmless enough, but has Jerry considered the possibility that the resident may not want others to have this information about his status?

In the second case, the DON is obviously concerned about breaking confidentiality to convey information to the children of a resident who is still fully competent mentally. But there is also a more subtle issue of confidentiality; namely, whether it was appropriate for the housekeeper to report to the DON that this resident had in his possession a drug prescribed to enhance sexual potency. Finally, the resident's physician alludes to the practice of confidentiality in saying that "such a prescription is a matter solely between a doctor and his patient."

Why Confidentiality Is a Value in Health Care

Confidentiality is an important value for several reasons. If confidentiality is not maintained by health care workers, then individuals may be deterred from seeking treatment they need. Further, if confidentiality is not maintained, they may not want to disclose all the information that is necessary for adequate treatment. This is because some medical problems are quite personal, such as sexual dysfunction. Some diseases carry a social stigma, such as AIDS and mental illness. Some people may feel embarrassed by open discussion of their bodily functions. Some people are simply more private than others about what is going on with them. And, legally, we do recognize a *right to privacy*.

To appreciate the value of confidentiality, just consider what appears on the evening news when the President of the United States or another prominent person has a serious health problem and must have surgery or other treatment. Would you want this kind of information broadcast about yourself?

The Principle of Confidentiality

As an ethical principle, there is a strong prima facie obligation to maintain confidentiality about medical information. In others words, *there is an expectation that confidentiality be maintained about medical information, unless the value of maintaining confidentiality is overridden by exceptional circumstances.* The exceptional circumstances that are recognized to justify breaking confidentiality are *preventing serious harm from coming to other people, or to the patient/resident.* (2, 3)

As concerned as Irma Todd may be about her neighbor and friend, Larry Steffen, and however harmless it may seem for Jerry Miller, the CNA, to give her a progress report on Larry's condition, it is not ethically right for Jerry to do so. Health care workers are expected to maintain confidentiality about the medical status of patients and residents they care for and about information learned in the course of their work. Jerry's breach of confidentiality is not justified on grounds of preventing harm to anyone. Health care workers need to be very careful about the kind of mistake Jerry Miller made, which is an easy one to make. It is good if they have in mind some polite responses to the kind of inquiry posed by Irma Todd that will not give out medical information. For example, Jerry might say something like this: "My contact with Larry is limited. Why don't you come to visit him and see for yourself ?" This kind of response would respect Larry's wishes by giving him the prerogative of deciding what medical information he does and does not want to share with neighbors.

Concomitantly, health care facilities and services should emphasize confidentiality as a job expectation of everyone involved in patient and resident care, whether directly or indirectly, and no matter what his or her particular job is. In fact, it has been suggested that job descriptions for health care workers should explicitly mention respect for confidentiality among job qualifications and that one standard by which a health care worker's job performance should be evaluated is his demonstrated respect for patient confidentiality. (4) This recommendation is reinforced by the governmental HIPAA privacy regulations (see below).

Ethically, confidentiality may be broken to prevent serious harm from coming to other people, or (some would add) to the patient or resident herself. What might be some examples where these exceptions to confidentiality apply? A psychologist treating an individual who threatens to kill a specific, identifiable person may be justified in breaking confidentiality to warn the intended victim (and indeed, legally expected to do so). (5) Similarly, breaking confidentiality may be necessary in the case of involuntary commitment proceedings for an individual who is apt to commit suicide or engage in self-mutilating behavior. This breach of confidentiality falls into the category of preventing serious harm to the patient or resident himself. Legally, health care workers may be required to report cases of child abuse, gunshot and knife wounds, and cases of communicable disease. The last requirement is clearly an instance of trying to prevent harm to other people. The requirements to report cases of child abuse and gunshot and knife wounds may fall into both categories; namely, preventing further harm to the present victim and preventing the same harm from being inflicted on yet other people.

In the second case scenario, there clearly is the danger of significant harm to other people posed by the male resident possessing a drug to enhance sexual potency. It is entirely possible that he could entrap female residents suffering from dementia into having sexual relations with him. Thus, from an ethical point of view, it seems that the housekeeper was entirely justified in alerting the DON to his possession of the drug. It also seems that the DON would be justified in breaking confidentiality about medical information in order to inform the resident's children about their father's possession of the drug in the hope they will persuade him to relinquish it. In reaching this judgment, however, it is important to note that other ways of handling the situation were tried first, and failed. The director of nursing tried to speak both to the resident and to the resident's physician, but this did not resolve the problem.

It should be emphasized that breaches of confidentiality are exceptional cases. Apart from legally mandated reporting requirements, health care workers should be extremely cautious about breaking confidentiality. In the vast majority of cases, confidentiality about medical information remains the rule.

Confidentiality and Computerized Health Information

The confidentiality of medical records is an area of major concern today. On one level, there is always concern that health care workers are careful about where they put medical charts so that unauthorized persons may not see them. But a significant challenge today lies in the placement of medical records on computer. Along with this, there is concern about the development of "health information networks" that allow the electronic exchange of financial and clinical information among the various components of the health care system, including hospitals, physicians, pharmacists, other health care providers, payers, and employers. (4)

Putting medical records on computer has distinct advantages, not only for the acute care setting but also for long-term care. Individuals can be transferred from a hospital to a long-term care facility or from a long-term care facility to a hospital. Computerized medical records facilitate the transfer of needed information between the two facilities, especially when a resident is taken to a hospital emergency room. (6) Indeed, emergency room physicians have noted "problems in obtaining information about elderly nursing home residents in up to three-quarters of all cases..." (6) Computerized medical records can also lead to better care for residents in other ways. One study reported "a significant decrease in urinary incontinence among nursing home patients whose care plan was developed with the assistance of a computerized expert nurse system." (6) Computerized records can improve care through "computer programs such as software to monitor drug-drug interactions, computer-generated alerts and reminders, and on-line consultation." (7)

At the same time, there are problems and abuses that have occurred with computerized medical records and the development of health information networks. (4, 8) In one case, the teenaged daughter of a hospital emergency room clerk printed out the names and telephone numbers of patients who had used the emergency room the previous weekend, called them, and falsely told them that they were either pregnant or HIV positive. One of those contacted attempted suicide. (4) In another incident, Medicaid clerks tapped into computers and printed out patient names, addresses, incomes, and medical records and sold them to recruiters for health maintenance organizations (HMOs). (4) Potential abuses in the electronic transmission of health care information are motivating factors behind the enactment of the HIPAA regulations. (9)

HIPAA Regulations

In 1996 the United States Congress enacted the Health Insurance Portability and Accountability Act (HIPAA). In addition to requirements concerning the transferability of health insurance, this legislation provides a comprehensive framework for regulating the standardization, security, and privacy of health information. The HIPAA statute as such focuses on the electronic exchange of health information. However, as implemented by the U.S. Department of Health and Human Services, HIPAA regulations are much broader and govern essentially all collection, maintenance, transmission, use, and disclosure of "individually identifiable health information." The regulations address standards for transactions (such as health claims and health care payments) to enable the electronic interchange of health information, for a unique health identifier for each individual, for code sets for appropriate data elements for transactions, for security of health information, for electronic signatures, for transfer of information among health plans, and for privacy. (9) The privacy standards in particular interface with the ethical issue of confidentiality.

The U.S. Office for Civil Rights has offered the following rationale for the development of the privacy standards:

> Under the current patchwork of laws, personal health information can be distributed—without either notice or consent—for reasons that have nothing to do with a patient's medical treatment or health care reimbursement. Patient information held by a health plan may be passed on to a lender who may then deny the patient's application for a home mortgage or a credit card—or to an employer who may use it in personnel decisions. The Privacy Rule establishes a federal floor of safeguards to protect the confidentiality of medical information. (10)

According to the Office for Civil Rights, the Privacy Rule "gives patients more control over their health information" and enables them "to make informed choices when seeking care and reimbursement for care based on how personal health information may be used." (10) This is in line with the ethical emphasis on individual autonomy—that is, directing the course of one's own life. At the same time, the Privacy Rule recognizes situations where *public responsibility* requires disclosure of some forms of data—for example, to protect public health." (10) Such exceptions are in line with the ethical principle of confidentiality, which allows disclosure of information to prevent significant harm from coming to other persons.

As evidenced by the ethical principle of confidentiality, discussions of confidentiality have traditionally focused on the *disclosure* of information. However, the HIPAA Privacy Rule includes as well the *use* of health care information. (9) It has also refined the ethical concept of informed consent in "laying out several different levels or types of consent or authorization that must be obtained, depending on the purpose of the intended use or disclosure" (9):

> Uses or disclosures for treatment, payment or health care operations will require a basic, relatively simple signed "consent," while many other uses and disclosures will require a more detailed "authorization." Still other uses or disclosures, such as being listed in a facility directory, require only that the individual be given notice with the opportunity to reject. (9)

The HIPAA Privacy Rule has defined a set of legal rights for patients and residents: a right to be informed about a health care facility's privacy practices, a right to request restrictions on the use or disclosure of health information, a right to obtain access to protected health information for inspection and copying, a right to an accounting of disclosures of health information, and a right to request amendments to health care records. Moreover, following a "need to know" principle, the Privacy Rule specifies that health care facilities must make reasonable efforts "to use, disclose or request only the minimum amount of protected health information necessary to accomplish the intended purpose of the use or disclosure." (9)

The Privacy Rule includes stipulations covering a broad spectrum of activities, persons, and organizations. It covers treatment, payment, marketing, fundraising, research, and relations with vendors and service providers (e.g., pharmacies, software vendors). It affects how admissions and transfers are to be handled, as well as computer terminals and faxing. It covers information provided to accrediting agencies, such as the Joint Commission on Accreditation of Healthcare Organizations (JCAHO). It impacts how oral communications among staff members are to be handled. It impacts information that can be given to members of the facility's Board of Trustees, clergy, and even family members and close friends of residents. (9) The stipulations of the Privacy Rule may seem unwarrantedly detailed, onerous, and just another example of governmental bureaucracy. From a more positive perspective, they can be viewed as an attempt to raise our consciousness about the many arenas in which the ethical principle of confidentiality has applicability.

FOR GROUP DISCUSSION

1. Consider the case of Jerry Miller at the beginning of this chapter. Suppose that he had met the pastor of Larry Steffen's church at the grocery store and that the pastor had inquired about Larry's condition. Should this make any difference in the way in which Jerry should respond to the inquiries about Larry's condition?

2. Ted Martin works as a physical therapist at Mercy Medical Center, but also provides services to several area nursing homes, including Crestridge Manor. One of Mercy's patients, Darlene Tucker, 79, is about to be transferred to Crestridge. Darlene was hospitalized for a broken hip but, while in the hospital, it was discovered that she also had an infection. The infection proved resistant to antibiotics. At present, the infection has taken its course and Darlene has recovered from it, but the infection could recur later.

   Ted Martin has treated Darlene while at Mercy and knows about her antibiotic resistant infection since he had to take special precautions for infection control while giving her physical therapy. Crestridge Manor has agreed to accept Darlene as a resident without seeing her complete medical record. Ted knows that, up to this time, the staff of Crestridge has not had to deal with a resident subject to antibiotic resistant infections. He worries that the staff at Crestridge is not properly trained in the infection control procedures needed to prevent the spread of antibiotic resistant organisms, and that many other residents could be adversely affected if Darlene becomes a resident at Crestridge and the infection recurs. Especially since he is effectually part-time at Crestridge, Ted wonders if he should take the initiative of informing the administrator of Crestridge about Darlene's antibiotic resistant infection before she is transferred there from the hospital.

   From an ethical point of view, should Ted Martin break confidentiality and inform Crestridge Manor of Darlene's recent antibiotic resistant infection? What are the pros of breaking confidentiality? The cons? Is there any way in which Ted can handle this situation without breaking confidentiality?

3. Rita Barton works as an RN at the Four Oaks Home. One afternoon at the nursing station she receives a call from the physician of a resident, Tom Morton, to inquire about how Tom is tolerating a new medication for depression. Physicians are busy people, so Rita has to be open in discussing Tom's condition with the physician on the spot. However, several other residents who are passing by the nurses' station overhear parts of the conversation, including mention of Tom by name.

   Tom likes to attend chapel services when a local pastor comes to Four Oaks on Wednesdays. However, this new medication occasionally makes him dizzy. For this reason, Rita Barton escorts Tom to the chapel. She also makes a point of telling the CNA (certified nursing assistant) on duty in the chapel to keep an eye on Tom for dizzy spells due to his medication.

   • Evaluate how Rita handled the telephone call at the nurses' station from the perspective of confidentiality. Are there any alternative ways in which this situation could have been handled?

   • From the perspective of maintaining confidentiality about resident health information, how should communications between staff members regarding residents be conducted in public areas of the facility (like a chapel)?

4. A nursing student at a local college is interested in music therapy. This student approaches the administrator of the Four Oaks Home about conducting a

research project for a course in geriatric nursing she is taking. The research project will consist in playing selected pieces of classical music to agitated residents to determine if the music has a calming effect on them. The student will write a paper on this research project and its outcome for her class. What kind of information about the individual residents who participate in this research project should the student be allowed to include in her class paper?

5. Providing medical treatment for a resident sometimes involves looking at ethical questions and consulting with a facility's ethics committee. Suppose there is a controversy among family members about insertion of a feeding tube into a resident in the Alzheimer's unit of the Four Oaks Home. Staff who are caring for this resident are also divided about what should be done. The Director of Nursing (DON) requests an ethics consult with the facility's ethics committee. The consult will involve herself and other members of the nursing staff but not the family—at least, not yet. The ethics committee includes both staff of the Four Oaks Home and people from the local community. What information about the resident should be disclosed to the ethics committee?

6. When the Four Oaks Home was built, the administrator's office was located near the main entrance in order to be visible and accessible to residents, family members, and those inquiring about admission to the facility. Outside the administrator's office is a small alcove that opens onto a large lounge area. Originally, this alcove was meant to be a reception area. However, because of a shortage of space at the facility, there are now three support staff persons with their desks and computers crowded into this area. A photocopier, a laser printer, and a fax machine, all shared by the administrator and the three support staff persons, have also been placed here. A pigeonhole mailbox unit for administrators and managers has been attached to one wall, and is used for internal communications as well as U.S. mail.

This office arrangement has already resulted in several situations that have left the administrator somewhat uneasy. On one occasion, two faxes arrived in succession. The first fax was intended for the business office and concerned billing for snow removal in the facility's parking lot. The second fax came from a physician's office, and contained information about possible side effects for a new medication that Harold Jones, a resident, was taking. A secretary picked up both of these faxes and gave them to the facility's accountant, who discovered the medical information and sent it to the nurses' station in Mr. Jones's wing.

On another occasion a group of school children was visiting with residents in the lounge area adjacent to this workspace. One boy, who is fascinated with computers, wandered over to an empty desk where the computer was on. Displayed on the screen was information from a resident's MDS (minimum data set). The secretary had temporarily left her desk in response to inquiries from a visitor trying to locate a resident's room.

Identify, in this office setting, other potential conditions for information about residents getting into the wrong hands. How might this workspace be rearranged to guard against unintentional breaches of confidentiality?

7. For each of the above scenarios, compare your response with what is specified by HIPAA privacy regulations.

NOTES

1. "Confidentiality" in Ronald Munson (ed.), *Intervention and Reflection Basic Issues in Medical Ethics*, 5th ed. (Belmont, CA: Wadsworth, 1996).
2. Tom L. Beauchamp & James F. Childress, *Principles of Biomedical Ethics* (New York: Oxford, 1979).
3. Benedict M. Ashley, OP & Kevin O'Rourke, OP, *Health Care Ethics*, 3rd ed. (St. Louis, MO: Catholic Health Association, 1989).
4. Ida Critelli Schick, "Protecting Patients' Privacy," *Health Progress* (May-June 1998): 26-31.
5. See California Supreme Court, *Tarasoff v. Regents of the University of California*, 131 California Reporter14 (July 1, 1976).
6. William Kavesh, "Integrated Communications Systems in Long-Term Care" in Paul R. Katz, Robert L. Kane, Mathy D. Mezey (eds.), *Quality Care in Geriatric Settings: Focus on Ethical Issues* (New York: Springer, 1995).
7. Jonathan S. Wald, "Computer-Based Patient Records," *New England Journal of Medicine* 334/17 (April 25, 1996): 1139.
8. Ross Anderson, "Clinical System Security: Interim Guidelines," *British Medical Journal* 312 (13 Jan. 1996): 109-11.
9. Maureen Weaver, Jeanette C. Schreiber, Michelle Wilcox DeBarge, Catherine P. Baatz, Wiggin & Dana, LLP, *The HIPAA Handbook Implementing the Federal Privacy Rule in the Long-Term Care Setting* (Washington, DC: American Association of Homes and Services for the Aging, 2001).
10. Office of Civil Rights, "Standards for Privacy of Individually Identifiable Health Information." http://www.hhs.gov/ocr/hipaa/finalmaster.html

FOR FURTHER STUDY

• Thomas A. Mappes and David DeGrazia (eds.), *Biomedical Ethics*, 4th ed. (New York: McGraw-Hill, 1996), Chapter 3, subsection on Confidentiality. This subsection contains four readings, including the court decision in the Tarasoff case.

• Audrey R. Chapman, *Health Care and Information Ethics* (Kansas City, MO: Sheed & Ward, 1997).

• Maureen Weaver, Jeanette C. Schreiber, Michelle Wilcox DeBarge, Catherine P. Baatz, Wiggin & Dana, LLP, *The HIPAA Handbook Implementing the Federal Privacy Rule in the Long-Term Care Setting* (Washington, DC: American Association of Homes and Services for the Aging, 2001).

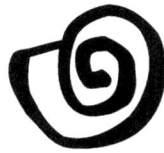

Chapter 15

Workplace Ethics

Some of the chapters in this book discuss ethical dilemmas faced by residents and their families. Should tube feeding be started for a resident who has suffered a severe stroke? When should a do-not-resuscitate order be in place for an elderly patient with Alzheimer's disease? Is it morally permissible for a father suffering from a progressively debilitating disease to commit suicide?

This chapter will have a different focus. It will examine the moral responsibilities of health care workers themselves and ethical dilemmas that they may face as *employees* of a health care facility.

This chapter covers:
* *ethical reasons for regularly coming to work;*
* *the ethics of health care workers "using their own judgment" in going against treatment orders for residents they are caring for;*
* *a health care worker's moral responsibilities when a co-worker isn't doing his or her job.*

CASE STUDY

Brigid O'Connor is Director of Nursing at the Spring Valley Home. Among her duties she is responsible for seeing that there is adequate staffing. On several occasions she has called in Sally Furtweiler, one of the certified nursing assistants (CNAs). Sally frequently calls in at the last minute that she cannot come to work that day. On one occasion she said she had car trouble. On another occasion she had an emergency dental appointment. On more than one occasion she's said that she cannot come to work because of a sick child or because of bad weather. Then there was the time that Sally's sister came to visit her from California. Brigid is tempted to fire Sally for excessive absenteeism, but she doesn't do so because of the shortage of CNAs at nursing homes in the area. Brigid reasons that having a CNA part of the time is better than none!

However, Sally being absent from work unexpectedly and frequently does present a staffing problem. Ruth is the CNA who works with Sally on the same wing and shift, and Ruth has complained to Brigid several times about not being able to take care of all the residents properly when Sally is absent. Ruth finds herself having to make choices about which residents should receive attention and which ones will just have to make due without her. On the day that Sally stayed home because her sister came to visit her from California, Ruth started to assist a female resident, Millie, with getting dressed up for family coming to visit her from some distance. Millie has always been very meticulous about her personal appearance, but she now needs considerable help with dressing because of swollen legs and severe arthritis.

Ruth felt an obligation to spend time with Millie to help her look her best for her family since she knows how important this is to her.

However, while Ruth was helping Millie, another resident, Alice, turned on the call light for assistance in going to the bathroom. Alice has problems with incontinence, and she is very self-conscious about having an accident in her bed. She finds it very offensive to her dignity "to have to be cleaned up like a baby." Ruth is aware of this, and usually tries hard to answer Alice's call light quickly.

Ruth also had to watch John. John is suffering from dementia, and when he takes walks in the hall, he sometimes forgets where his room is. He wanders into the rooms of other residents and yells at them to "get out of his room." Several of the women residents are terrified of John because he has tried to physically drag them out of their rooms. And amidst all of this another resident, Henry, started choking on a piece of candy he wasn't supposed to have in the first place!

The Duty to Come to Work

We would all agree that there are emergency situations that make absence from work necessary and justified. However, it seems that Sally Furtweiler is not taking her "duty to come to work" seriously enough. She frequently calls in at the last minute to say she will not be at work. She cannot even manage to coordinate the visit of a sister from California with her work schedule.

From an ethical point of view, exactly what grounds are there for claiming that Sally (or anyone, for that matter) has a moral obligation to show up for work? This claim can be backed up in several ways.

First of all, it is recognized that we have a duty to keep promises. Employment is a type of contract in which the employee promises to provide certain services to the employer and the employer in turn promises certain wages and benefits to the employee. By her frequent absences Sally is breaking the promise she made to the Spring Valley Home when she accepted employment there.

Moreover, health care ethicists recognize a *principle of nonmaleficence*: the duty of a health care worker to prevent harm from coming to residents. If Spring Valley Home has a CNA staffing shortage on a particular shift because Sally does not come to work, there is the potential that residents may suffer harm. Resident Henry may choke on the piece of hard candy because CNA Ruth is busy with other residents and does not notice that this is happening. Women residents may suffer the psychological harm of being scared by John when he mistakenly wanders into their rooms and tries to evict them.

One approach to ethical theory is the *consequentialist* approach. As the name indicates, a consequentialist theory judges rightness and wrongness of actions by their consequences. One type of consequentialist theory is *utilitarianism*. A utilitarian considers consequences for everyone to be affected by an action. According to a utilitarian, the right action to perform is the one that will have the best consequences overall when everyone to be affected by the action is taken into account. Utilitarianism can also establish that Sally has a duty to go to work.

Consider, for example, the case of Sally deciding to stay home from work when her sister visits her from California. For Sally, the course of action of staying home from work will have the good consequence of giving her more time to spend with her sister (although it will also have the negative consequence for Sally of losing a day's pay). But what about the other people who will be affected? Sally staying home from work will have the negative consequence of making CNA Ruth's shift very pressured and stressful for her. Sally staying home from work is likely to have some negative consequences for the residents on her wing of the Spring Valley Home. For lack of adequate staffing, Alice may experience the indignity of having an accident in her bed. Millie may feel uncomfortable and embarrassed when her family comes to visit her because her appearance isn't what she wants it to be. John's unsupervised wandering may result in some of the women residents becoming scared and apprehensive. On balance, it clearly seems that the good consequences for Sally of staying home from work to be with her sister are outweighed by many negative consequences for other people. Overall, the consequences of Sally failing to go to work are bad, so this cannot be the right action to perform by utilitarian standards.

CASE STUDY

Julie Ames works as a dietitian at Spring Valley Home. Part of her job is making sure that dietary restrictions for particular residents are observed. Because of heart problems, George Mason's doctor has put him on a low-fat, low sodium diet. George usually cooperates without too much complaint, but he does love sweet corn and "just can't eat it without some salt." Spring Valley always has a picnic for residents on the Fourth of July, and this year a local farmer—in fact, a friend of George—has donated a truckload of sweet corn to the home for the picnic. Julie knows that George will really feel left out and hurt if he isn't served sweet corn, especially since it comes from a personal friend. She also knows that if George is served the sweet corn plain, he will raise a fuss with the staff about getting some salt. And a conflict between George and the staff during the picnic will ruin the day for both him and the staff. Julie decides to slip two packets of salt onto George's tray. After all, George's doctor will never know, and this one breach of his diet shouldn't harm him.

Staff Who "Use Their Own Judgment"

In this case, a staff member of a health care facility takes it upon herself to do something for a resident that directly goes against the orders of a physician. The staff member makes the judgment that going against the physician's orders will not harm the resident's health. Ethically, is it permissible for staff to act in this way?

Some would approach this case not by looking at the behavior of staff, but rather by focusing on residents and their autonomy. Allowing a person to direct the course of his or her own life is a value much emphasized in contemporary health care ethics. Thus, some would argue that the proper course of action is to explain to

George the possible consequences for his heart condition of using salt, but to allow him to make the decision whether he wishes to take those risks. Once health care providers have informed George of the risks and are confident that he understands them and is mentally competent to make decisions, then both the physician and the nursing home staff should abide by George's wishes, even if they personally disagree with his choice. Thus, if George wants salt for his sweet corn, he should have it! (1)

However, not everyone would place such an exclusive emphasis on patient autonomy. They would point out that health care providers have a duty of *nonmaleficence*, that is, a duty to prevent harm from coming to residents. In the case of George, autonomy and nonmaleficence may be in conflict. In others words, there may be a conflict between what George wants to do in terms of eating and what his doctor believes should be done to prevent further harm to his already fragile health.

The question can be raised whether Julie the dietitian violated the ethical duty of nonmaleficence in providing salt for George. She "used her own judgment" in believing that George would not be harmed by her action. But can she really be so sure that she has the professional knowledge to make these assessments on her own?

Further, Julie's behavior is ethically questionable because it is deceptive. In slipping two packets of salt onto George's tray, Julie believes that "George's doctor will never know."

If staff member Julie questioned the wisdom of an absolute prohibition of salt seasoning for George, it would have been more appropriate for her to raise this question with her supervisor, with George's physician, or at the care conference for George. Bringing this question out into the open would provide the opportunity to discuss whether occasional indulgences in salt seasoning would in fact be harmful to George's health. After discussion, perhaps his physician would agree to occasional indulgences.

CASE STUDY

Rhonda Lewis is an RN who has worked for ten years at Spring Valley Home. She is known as a good worker and as someone who is very conscientious. Rhonda has some concerns about Jerry Miles who comes every week to administer physical therapy to some of the residents of Spring Valley Home. Several times, she has smelled alcohol on Jerry's breath. On one occasion she walked into George Mason's room and found Jerry helping him with exercises for his legs. The problem is that George didn't need these exercises. Jerry was supposed to give them to the man in the room next to George's. George wasn't at all hurt by this mistake, but Rhonda wonders how often this kind of mistake is occurring. Another resident, Henry Thompson, has complained to her that Jerry has skipped him on several occasions. And when Henry doesn't get his exercises, he gets stiff and experiences some difficulty in walking. Rhonda wonders what she should do. She has always believed that co-workers should not "rat" on each other. And she knows how difficult it is to get outside health care workers to provide services at a nursing home, especially on a weekly basis.   What will the residents of Spring Valley Home do if they lose Jerry?

Problems with the Job Performance of Co-Workers

In this case, Rhonda is concerned about the job performance of a co-worker, Jerry, who comes to Spring Valley Home to administer physical therapy to some of the residents. She has caught one mistake Jerry made on the job, giving exercises to the wrong resident. In this case, the mistake didn't cause the resident any harm. But if this sort of mistake occurs again, it is possible that Jerry could give exercises to a resident who would suffer muscular or bone damage. Also, Jerry has caused discomfort to another resident on several occasions by forgetting about his therapy altogether. In addition, Rhonda worries about the fact that she has smelled alcohol on Jerry's breath several times. She knows that alcohol can impair performance, and cause someone to make mistakes.

The moral duty of nonmaleficence tells Rhonda that she must act to prevent harm from coming to the residents of Spring Valley Home. The situation with Jerry presents the potential for harm. Therefore, Rhonda cannot just let this situation slip by, but is morally obligated to take action.

Rhonda has strong feelings that co-workers should not "rat" on each other. Perhaps, then, the first step is for Rhonda to confront Jerry with her concerns about his job performance. Is it the case that Jerry has made mistakes and been forgetful because of a stressful situation within his own family that is only temporary? Or are his mistakes and forgetfulness due to a more enduring problem? And what is the cause of Jerry's apparent alcohol abuse? On his own, will Jerry decide to get appropriate professional help if needed?

In her job, Rhonda's first obligation is to the residents of Spring Valley Home and to promoting their welfare and protecting them from harm.   If Rhonda's conversation with Jerry does not result in a change of job performance, or if Rhonda does not feel comfortable about having such a conversation with Jerry, then she has an obligation to report this situation to her supervisor. While she may not want to "rat" on Jerry, her obligation to prevent harm to residents takes precedence over her feelings.

FOR GROUP DISCUSSION

1. There may be bad consequences for residents and other health care workers when someone fails to show up for work. In what circumstances do you think it is legitimate for a health care worker to decide not to come to work? Is bad weather a legitimate reason? Caring for a sick child? Personal illness? An emergency dental appointment? (Try using the utilitarian ethical theory in working through these questions, looking at the consequences for everyone who will be affected by the health care worker's action.)

2. Jeanette Taylor, 80, was admitted to the Spring Valley Home five days ago under its hospice program. It is known by the staff that Jeanette does not want

resuscitation attempts undertaken should she suffer an arrest. However, the Director of Nursing has not yet gotten the physician's do-not-resuscitate (DNR) order written in her medical chart because Jeanette's doctor has been out of town on vacation for the last week.

Darlene Zimmerman is the supervising nurse on the late shift. At 2:00 a.m. she goes into Jeanette's room to check on her, and finds that she has arrested. Darlene knows that state regulations require her to undertake cardiopulmonary resuscitation unless the resident has a written DNR order. At the same time, she knows that Jeanette is dying and doesn't want to be resuscitated. Darlene has always considered herself to be someone who advocates for the wishes of the resident when it comes to end-of-life treatment decisions.

There is no one else around, as the CNAs are on break. Darlene decides to use her own judgment about the right thing to do in this case. She walks out of Jeanette's room, and does not return until half an hour later. At this time she calls in one of the CNAs and announces that Jeanette has died in her sleep. They begin the arrangements to remove the body and to notify Jeanette's family of her death.

In your judgment, did Darlene do the right thing in using her own judgment and acting against state regulations by not undertaking cardiopulmonary resuscitation on Jeanette? On what considerations and principles do you base your judgment?

3. Ted Collins is on the dietary staff at Spring Valley Home. He smokes heavily. He doesn't smoke in the facility itself, but whenever he gets a break from his work in the kitchen, he goes outside and lights up. A co-worker, Jill Pierce, is upset with Ted for doing this. She tells him that residents who are walking or sitting outdoors can see him smoke, and that this tempts residents who are restricted from smoking for health reasons. Jill tells her supervisor that Ted should be made to give up smoking entirely while at work.

   • Is this situation different than the case of Jerry Miles who showed up at Spring Valley Home to administer physical therapy with alcohol on his breath?

   • Jill's complaints to her supervisor would be legitimate and would fall under the duty of nonmaleficence if Ted's behavior at work poses a threat of harm to the residents. Can a case be made that Ted is harming residents by his smoking?

4. Suppose that you are asked to serve on an ad hoc committee to develop specific criteria for the annual staff evaluation process. What specific standards would you suggest for the areas of absence from work, following treatment directives for residents, and handling job performance problems with co-workers? And why would you suggest these particular standards?

NOTES

1. "Beyond the Call of Duty: A Nurse's Aide Uses Her Judgment," in Rosalie Kane & Arthur L. Caplan (eds.), *Everyday Ethics Resolving Dilemmas in Nursing Home Life* (New York: Springer, 1990).

FOR FURTHER STUDY

- Rosalie A. Kane and Arthur L. Caplan (eds.), *Everyday Ethics Resolving Dilemmas in Nursing Home Life* (New York: Springer, 1990), chapters 17, 20. Case studies with commentary.

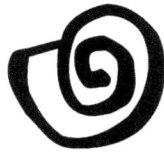

Chapter 16

Moral and Religious Objections to Medical Practices

Health care practices can be morally and religiously controversial. The abortion debate in the United States is a prime example of this. Some people favor assisted suicide, whereas others are opposed to it on moral and religious grounds. Some have objections in conscience to such practices as artificial insemination, in vitro fertilization, and the freezing of embryos. While most people in American society take blood transfusions for granted, Jehovah's Witnesses refuse them on religious grounds.

Patients will bring their moral and religious values with them when seeking health care services. Similarly, health care workers also have personal beliefs about what is right and wrong to do.

This chapter covers:
* *the right of an adult to refuse a medical treatment on moral or religious grounds;*
* *the right of a health care worker to be excused from participating in a treatment or course of action to which he has moral or religious objections.*

CASE STUDY

Rebecca Schmidt, 77, has been a resident of St. Ann's Home, a multi-level facility, for two years. She has difficulty and pain in walking, and her doctor has suggested both knee and hip replacement surgeries. She remains very alert mentally, and is known among the staff of St. Ann's as a great conversationalist.

Recently it was discovered that Rebecca has stomach cancer. Chemotherapy has been started, and the prospects for the cancer going into remission look fairly good. However, because of the bleeding caused by the presence of the tumor, Rebecca has become anemic and needs blood transfusions to assist in her recovery.

When Rebecca is approached about beginning the transfusions, she unqualifiedly refuses. She states that she is a Jehovah's Witness, and that her religion does not permit blood transfusions. She says she will put her faith in God. "If God wants me to continue to live," she states, "I will recover without the blood transfusions."

St. Ann's Home is a Catholic-sponsored facility, a religious tradition that accepts the practice of blood transfusions. The staff at St. Ann's cannot understand how there can be *religious* reasons for refusing a blood transfusion that will be clearly beneficial to someone's health. Rebecca has become especially fond of Marge Malone, the activity director at St. Ann's, and several staff members ask Marge to talk to Rebecca about the transfusions. Marge poses to Rebecca a situation in which she thinks it will be impossible for Rebecca to condemn transfusions. "Think back to the time when your son was just five years old," Marge tells Rebecca, "and was injured in an automobile accident. Suppose that your son had been so severely injured that he would die unless he had a blood transfusion. As a mother, wouldn't you have wanted the transfusion to save your son's life?" To Marge's surprise, Rebecca calmly replies that she could have accepted her son's death as God's will.

At this point, Marge and several other staff members ask to meet with St. Ann's ethics committee to help them work through this baffling situation.

Objections to Medical Practice by Residents and Families

Perhaps the classic case of a religious objection to a medical practice is the refusal of blood transfusions by Jehovah's Witnesses. This refusal is based on biblical texts, such as Genesis 9:4, Leviticus 3:17 and 7:26, and Acts 15:28-29 which forbid "partaking of any blood." (1, 2)

A famous court case involving the refusal of blood transfusions by a Jehovah's Witness is *In re Brooks Estate* from the state of Illinois. In May 1964, Bernice Brooks was in McNeal General Hospital in Chicago, suffering from a peptic ulcer. She was attended by Dr. Gilbert Demange, and had informed him repeatedly during a two-year period prior to her hospitalization that her religious beliefs prevented her from receiving blood transfusions. In fact, Mrs. Brooks and her husband signed a document releasing Dr. Demange and the hospital from all civil liability that might result from a failure to administer blood transfusions to Mrs. Brooks. In spite of this, Dr. Demange, together with several assistant State's attorneys and the attorney for the public guardian of Cook County, Illinois, appeared before the probate division of the circuit court with a petition by the public guardian requesting appointment of the guardian as "conservator" of Bernice Brooks. Further, the petition requested an order authorizing the conservator to consent to administration of blood to Mrs. Brooks. The court appointed the conservator, and a blood transfusion was administered to Mrs. Brooks. (3)

This situation involved a conflict between what the patient wanted (namely, no blood transfusions) and what the physician felt obligated to do for the welfare of the patient. Ethically speaking, this situation involved a conflict between *patient autonomy* and the health care professional's duty of *beneficence*.

The Illinois court made the following judgment in this case:

> ...It seems to be clearly established that the First Amendment of the United States Constitution, as extended to the individual States by the Fourteenth Amendment to that Constitution, protects the absolute right of every individual to freedom in his religious belief and the exercise thereof, subject only to the qualification that the exercise thereof may be properly limited by governmental action where such exercise endangers, clearly and presently, the public health, welfare or morals.

...No overt or affirmative act of appellants offers any clear and present danger to society—we have only a governmental agency compelling conduct offensive to appellants' religious principles. Even though we may consider appellant's beliefs unwise, foolish or ridiculous, in the absence of an overriding danger to society we may not permit interference therewith in the form of a conservatorship established in the waning hours of her life for the sole purpose of compelling her to accept medical treatment forbidden by her religious principles and previously refused by her with full knowledge of the probable consequences. In the final analysis, what has happened here involves a judicial attempt to decide what course of action is best for a particular individual, notwithstanding that individual's contrary views based upon religious convictions. Such action cannot be constitutionally countenanced. (3)

The Illinois court took the position that an individual's religious freedom must be respected and can only be limited when the person's behavior threatens harm to society. Thus, Mrs. Brooks had the right to refuse blood transfusions on religious grounds, and it was wrong for a conservator to have been appointed to force blood transfusions on her.

In the case of Mrs. Brooks, the Illinois court came down on the side of patient autonomy. In general, it is recognized today that a mentally competent adult patient who has been adequately informed of the potential advantages and risks of a proposed treatment does have the right to refuse it, even when the best medical opinion deems it essential to save the person's life. (4, 5)

In sum, what would the ethics committee of St. Ann's Home say to Marge and the other staff members about the case of Rebecca Schmidt? From a legal point of view, it may well be judged that Rebecca has the prerogative to refuse the blood transfusions if the case is taken to court. Ethically, this case involves a conflict between two principles: the principle of autonomy (what the resident wants) and the principle of beneficence (what health care workers see as treatment necessary to promote the welfare of the resident). Thus, we must decide which ethical principle takes precedence in this case. Given the direction of contemporary health care ethics, it is fair to say that a number of persons would come down on the side of autonomy. In fact, standards for long-term care from the Joint Commission on Accreditation of Healthcare Organizations (JCAHO) affirm that "the resident has a right to considerate care that respects his or her personal values, beliefs, cultural and spiritual preferences, and life-long patterns of living" [RI.2.1]. (6) Several considerations might be brought forward to support giving priority to individual autonomy in this case.

First, patients other than Jehovah's Witnesses can and do make the choice not to follow their physician's recommendations. In one study, "19% of patients at teaching hospitals refused at least one treatment or procedure, even though 15% of such refusals were potentially life endangering." (7) Generalizing this point, refusing a medical procedure on religious grounds can be seen as one instance of the phenomenon of patient choice regarding medical treatments.

Moreover, there are other cases in which therapies have to be altered to accommodate special circumstances, such as hypertension, severe allergy to antibiotics, or the unavailability of certain costly equipment. (7) Analogously, when a patient objects to a particular medical treatment on religious grounds, health care providers "are being asked to manage the medical or surgical problem in harmony with the patient's choice and conscience." (7)

Finally, health care providers should keep in mind the psychological damage that may be inflicted on a patient by forcing her to undergo a medical treatment against her conscience:

> If a court forced an abhorrent treatment on you, how might this affect your conscience and the vital element of your will to live? Dr. Konrad Drebinger wrote: "It would certainly be a misguided form of medical ambition that would lead one to force a patient to accept a given therapy, overruling his conscience, so as to treat him physically but dealing his psyche a mortal blow. (2)

In other words, the focus should be on treating "the whole person." (8)

CASE STUDY

Terry Waters has recently received his BSN degree. His first job is at the Westfield Care Center. The administrator and director of nursing at Westfield are especially pleased to have Terry join the staff because of his interest in the field of gerontology. He has indicated a desire to pursue a master's degree in that field.

While in college Terry was very active in the campus pro-life group. He personally has strong feelings that it is morally wrong to withhold or withdraw life-sustaining treatments. This is, he believes, just a way of "getting rid of people who are difficult or whose care is expensive." He is also against advance directives because they can allow life-sustaining treatments to be forgone. In fact, he has a stack of pamphlets warning against advance directives, and during the first months of his employment at Westfield he has been seen passing them out to residents and family members.

Jack Springer is in the Alzheimer's unit at Westfield. He is in the final stages of the disease. A durable power of attorney for health care executed by Jack names his wife, Louise, as his proxy decision maker. Recently, Jack has developed pneumonia. After talking with their children, Louise tells Jack's physician that she doesn't want antibiotics given to Jack to try to treat his pneumonia. Alzheimer's disease is a terminal condition, she says, and Jack is at the stage where he can no longer enjoy life because he is bedridden and suffering from severe dementia. "Jack would never want to live like this," she states. It is time, she believes, that the natural dying process should be allowed to take its course. After all, pneumonia is "the old person's friend." Jack's physician agrees with her.

Terry is told that a decision has been made to forgo administering antibiotics to Jack and to provide only comfort care for him until he dies. The director of nursing (DON) tells Terry that they will rely heavily on him to provide this comfort care.

Since he is a graduate of a very good baccalaureate nursing program, he has had training in palliative care for the dying that some of the older nurses on staff lack. However, Terry tells the DON that Jack's family and physician are "killing him" by not administering antibiotics, and that his conscience will not allow him to be a part of this affair. "On moral grounds," he tells the DON, "I can no longer be involved in Jack's care."

Objections of Conscience by Health Care Workers

Health care workers may sometimes be in the position of being asked to perform a procedure or participate in a course of action to which they personally object on moral or religious grounds. A common case is the participation of health care workers in abortion procedures. But this is not the only kind of situation in which objections of conscience can arise. In this case, Terry, a new nurse, firmly believes it is morally wrong to withhold or withdraw life-sustaining treatments, and refuses to participate in the care of Jack Springer, a patient with pneumonia from whom antibiotics are being withheld by the choice of his proxy decision maker. In Terry's mind, continuing to participate in Jack's care while he is dying would be to participate in the process of deliberately causing a resident's death.

It is recognized that health care facilities can legitimately refuse to provide what a patient (or his proxy decision maker) may want. As stated by the Special Committee on Biomedical Ethics of the American Hospital Association, "Generally, a hospital may refuse to provide a service to a patient if the procedure is inappropriate to its mission (for example, therapeutic abortion, artificial insemination)." (9) Similarly, the federal *Patient Self-Determination Act* on advance directives contains a conscience clause. With respect to complying with the directives set out by a patient in a living will or durable power of attorney for health care, no facility is required to act contrary to its own mission and ethical values. However, a health care facility must have clearly written policies specifying the limits on the procedures it will perform, and make this information available to its clients. (10)

Similarly, it is recognized that health care workers have a right to refuse to participate in procedures and courses of action to which they personally have moral or religious objections. As stated by the Special Committee on Biomedical Ethics of the American Hospital Association:

> If a patient chooses a course of treatment that is not acceptable to the attending physician or other health care professionals, those individuals may withdraw from the case, as long as doing so does not amount to legal abandonment. If a suitably qualified alternative physician or health care professional willing to comply with the patient's preference is available, transfer to the care of that individual should be offered to the patient. (9)

Thus, if Terry believes it is morally wrong to withhold life-sustaining treatments (in this case, antibiotics for pneumonia), he should be allowed to withdraw from being involved in the care of Jack Springer, with another nurse taking his place. However, there are several provisos for this concession to Terry.

First, Terry has an obligation to make known his treatment refusal "in advance and in time for other appropriate arrangements to be made" for the care of the resident. (11) Terry knows that he has moral objections in principle to any case of withholding or withdrawing a life-sustaining treatment from a resident. And he knows that instances of withholding or withdrawing life-sustaining treatments are likely to occur in a nursing home setting. Thus, he has an obligation to let his supervisor know about his moral stance *before* he is faced with the case of Jack Springer. After all, the nursing home will have to make arrangements for someone else to take Terry's place in providing palliative care for Jack. If Terry just suddenly announces his moral objections to participating in Jack's care while he is dying, the nursing home may not be able to make staff reassignments quickly enough and Jack's dying process may turn out to be much more uncomfortable for him.

Second, Terry must make sure that his refusal to participate in Jack's care while dying is based on accurate and complete information. (11, 12) Terry believes that withholding or withdrawing life-sustaining treatments is just a way of "getting rid of people who are difficult or whose care is expensive." But does he really understand what people's motivation can be for forgoing life-sustaining treatments? The motivation of Jack's wife seems to be that she does not want to prolong her husband's suffering and that Jack himself would not want to live completely bedridden and with severe dementia. Does Terry recognize the emotional strain Jack's wife may be experiencing in "letting go" of her husband? Does Terry understand that there is a difference between forgoing life-sustaining treatments and involuntary euthanasia (which may be an attempt to "get rid of people")? Is he familiar with what ethicists and religious denominations are saying about the permissibility of forgoing life-sustaining treatments? In sum, before Terry can legitimately voice an objection of conscience to participating in Jack's care while he is dying, he has an obligation to become factually and ethically informed about withholding and withdrawing life-sustaining treatments.

Suppose that Terry persists in his belief that it is morally wrong to withhold or withdraw life-sustaining treatments. He may have to consider changing his place of employment. Apparently, it is a policy of Westfield Care Center to allow patients to forgo life-sustaining treatments. If it becomes a frequent occurrence that a substitute worker has to be found for Terry because of his objections of conscience and if this proves difficult for Terry's supervisor to do, then Terry's job performance may be called into question. In this case, it may be best for Terry to seek employment at a facility holding moral views more similar to his own. It is nothing new to say that there may be a price to pay for sticking to one's moral principles.

In dealing with the situation of objections of conscience by health care workers, there are obligations on the part of the health care facility as well as on the part of the worker. According to the standards for long-term care developed by the Joint Commission on Accreditation of Healthcare Organizations (JCAHO), a facility's policies and procedures should address how staff may request to be excused from participating in an aspect of resident care or treatment on grounds of conflicting cultural values, ethics, or religious beliefs and whether these factors are to be recognized as sufficient grounds for granting such requests [Intent of HR.5 and

HR.5.1]. (6) Further, a facility should have a written process defining the way such requests are managed [Intent of HR.5 and HR.5.1]. (6) Very importantly, the facility should have mechanisms in place to ensure that granting such a request will not negatively affect resident care or treatment [Intent of HR.5. and HR.5.1]. (6)

FOR GROUP DISCUSSION

1. Are there religious groups in your geographical area (e.g., Christian Scientists, Amish) whose religious beliefs may affect their acceptance of "standard" health care practices, procedures, and technologies? How much do you know about the beliefs of these groups?

2. Are there any procedures or courses of action in caring for residents that you personally find morally objectionable? Religiously objectionable? If so, what are the grounds on which you find them objectionable?

   Do you think your moral or religious views may cause you to run into any problems in your job or role in health care? Can you think of means to accommodate your objections of conscience while still doing your job or fulfilling your role satisfactorily?

3. If you are connected with a long-term care facility, critically review any policies the facility has in place to deal with moral and religious objections to procedures and practices on the part of residents or staff members. If no formal policies are in place, do you think any are needed? If so, what should be the content of these policies?

NOTES

1. Orville N. Griese, *Catholic Identity in Health Care: Principles and Practice* (Braintree, MA: Pope John Center, 1987).
2. Jehovah's Witnesses Official Web Site, "You Have the Right to Choose," http://www.watchtower.org/library/hb/article_04.htm
3. Emory C. Underwood, "From *In re Brooks Estate*" in J. Katz (ed.), *Experimentation with Human Beings* (New York: Russell Sage Foundation, 1972).
4. Laurance T. Wren, "Status of the Law on Medical and Religious Conflicts in Blood Transfusions," *Arizona Medicine* 24 (Oct. 1967): 970-3.
5. David H. Wilson, "Patients' Wishes Must Be Accepted," *British Medical Journal* 308 (28 May 1994): 1424.
6. Joint Commission on Accreditation of Healthcare Organizations, 2002-2003 *Standards for Long Term Care* (Oakbrook Terrace, IL: Joint Commission Resources, 2002).
7. J. Lowell Dixon, "Blood: Whose Choice and Whose Conscience?" *New York State Journal of Medicine* 88 (1988): 463-4.
8. "Jehovah's Witnesses: The Surgical/Ethical Challenge," *Journal of the American Medical Association* 246/21 (Nov. 27, 1981): 2471-2.

9. Special Committee on Biomedical Ethics, *Values in Conflict Resolving Ethical Issues in Hospital Care* (Chicago: American Hospital Association, 1985).
10. Catholic Health Association of the United States, *The Patient Self-Determination Act* (St. Louis: Catholic Health Association of the United States, 1991).
11. Ellen W. Bernal & Patricia S. Hoover, Commentary on "The Nurse's Appeal to Conscience" in Bette-Jane Crigger (ed.), *Cases in Bioethics Selections from the Hastings Center Report*, 3rd ed. (New York: St. Martin's Press, 1998).
12. Mila Ann Aroskar, Commentary on "The Nurse's Appeal to Conscience" in Bette-Jane Crigger (ed.), *Cases in Bioethics Selections from the Hastings Center Report*, 3rd ed. (New York: St. Martin's Press, 1998).

FOR FURTHER STUDY

• Peggy DesAutels, Margaret P. Battin and Larry May, *Praying for a Cure Medical Ethics in Conflict with Religious Freedom* (Boston: Rowman & Littlefield, 1998).

When the children of Christian Scientists die from a treatable illness, are their parents guilty of murder for withholding that treatment? How should the rights of children, the authority of the medical community, and religious freedom be balanced? Is it possible for those adhering to a medical model of health and disease and for those adhering to the Christian Science model to enter into a meaningful dialogue, or are the two models incommensurable? The authors of this book engage in a lucid and candid debate of the issues of who is ultimately responsible for deciding these questions and how to accommodate (and, in some cases, constrain) Christian Science views and practices within a pluralistic society.

• Stephen G. Post, "Baby K: Medical Futility and the Free Exercise of Religion," *Journal of Law, Medicine & Ethics* 23 (1995): 20-6.

• Rabbi Zev Schostak, "Jewish Ethical Guidelines for Resuscitation and Artificial Nutrition and Hydration of the Dying Elderly," *Journal of Medical Ethics* 20 (1994): 93-100.

• *Religious Traditions and Health Care Decisions Handbook Series* (Chicago: Park Ridge Center). Designed for health care workers, this series serves as a practical, easily accessible reference on the beliefs and moral positions of religious traditions regarding various clinical issues and procedures. Each handbook contains a historical synopsis, the tradition's fundamental beliefs about health care issues, and a discussion of the observances and practices that relate to care of the sick. Religious traditions represented in the series include Anabaptist, Buddhist, Christian Science, Episcopal, Islamic, Jehovah's Witness, Jewish, Latter-Day Saints, Lutheran, Orthodox Christian, Presbyterian, Roman Catholic, Seventh-Day Adventist, United Church of Christ, and United Methodist.

176 Chapter 16 • *Moral and Religious Objections*

- Leonard J. Weber, "When to Excuse Employees from Work Responsibilities," *Health Progress* 76/8 (Nov.-Dec. 1995): 50-1. This article includes proposed guidelines developed by the ethics committee of Mercy Hospital in Grayling, Michigan.

- Bette-Jane Crigger (ed.), *Cases in Bioethics Selections from the Hastings Center Report*, 3rd ed. (New York: St. Martin's Press, 1998), no. 2 "The Nurse's Appeal to Conscience" and no. 56 "My Conscience, Your Money."

- Kevin D. O'Rourke, O.P. and Philip Boyle, *Medical Ethics Sources of Catholic Teachings*, 3rd ed. (Washington, DC: Georgetown University Press, 1999), Chapter 2 "Formation of Conscience."

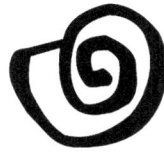

Chapter 17

Multicultural Perspectives on Health Care: The Case of Truth-Telling to the Terminally Ill

More and more it is being recognized that the principles of American health care ethicists may not be universally accepted. For example, Western health care ethics "endorses certain practices such as informed consent, disclosure of diagnosis and prognosis, and termination of treatment under certain conditions of terminal illness." (1) These practices, in turn, "reflect certain values widely held in Western culture: the autonomy of the individual person, the imperatives favoring truthfulness and open communication, and the realistic assessment of the efficacy of medical care." (1) However, health care workers who are trained in these practices and values may encounter patients and families from various cultures and subcultures who "react negatively or paradoxically to these practices." (1) In such cases conflicts can arise between health care providers and patients and their families.

This chapter will explore multiculturalism in health care through discussion of one particular issue involved in end-of-life care.

This chapter covers:
* *the practice of telling the truth about her condition to a patient who is terminally ill;*
* *cultures with different views from American culture on truth-telling, individual autonomy, and other health care practices;*
* *ways in which health care workers can deal with multiculturalism;*
* *the competing theories of ethical relativism and ethical absolutism.*

CASE STUDY

The Pleasant Hill Care Center is located in a Midwestern community that has recently seen an influx of Asian residents. This is because of a faculty and student exchange program established by the local college.

Mr. Chang has come with his family to the United States from China to teach at the college. Mr. Chang's mother, 84, accompanied them to the United States because she is a widow and in poor health. In fact, multiple health problems and general physical debilitation soon led to her placement in the Pleasant Hill Care Center.

The adjustment to the nursing home has been very difficult for Mrs. Chang, in part because she speaks very little English. Her son and daughter-in-law usually serve as interpreters for communications with the staff, but there are also some Chinese students from the college who visit the nursing home to converse with her.

Mrs. Chang becomes increasingly listless, and spends much of her time sleeping. When blood is discovered in her stools, she is sent to the hospital for diagnostic tests. The tests indicate that she has colon cancer, which has rapidly spread to other parts of her body. An oncologist, Marilyn Scott, tells her son that the cancer is "too far gone" for chemotherapy or surgery to be viable treatments. Dr. Scott recommends that measures be taken simply to keep her as comfortable as possible until she dies, most likely, in just a few months.

Dr. Scott asks Mr. Chang how his mother should be approached with this bad news. Mr. Chang insists that his mother be told absolutely nothing about her condition. He himself does not plan to tell her anything, and he virtually threatens Dr. Scott not to discuss anything with his mother through another interpreter.

Dr. Scott thinks that Mr. Chang's reaction comes from the initial shock of learning that his mother has a terminal illness. So she waits a few days, and then approaches him again. Mr. Chang reacts in precisely the same way. A week goes by, and Dr. Scott tries having another conversation with Mr. Chang but he remains adamant in his position.

Dr. Scott thinks that Mrs. Chang could profit from the hospice program available at the nursing home, but her son won't even listen to information about it. Dr. Scott also feels that a do-not-resuscitate order should be discussed with her.

Dr. Scott believes Mr. Chang is being unfair to his mother in not allowing her to be informed of her condition. After all, it's her life and it should be up to her to decide what treatments she does and does not want. Indeed, Dr. Scott has such negative feelings about the way in which Mr. Chang wants to handle the situation and his absolute refusal to agree to "standard medical practice" that she considers withdrawing from the case entirely.

Truth-Telling to the Terminally Ill

The case of Mrs. Chang concerns the ethical issue of telling the truth about a terminal condition to a patient. Her physician, Dr. Marilyn Scott, is concerned that she does not know her diagnosis and hence is unable to make her own decisions about the type and extent of treatment to receive as her life draws to a close. These concerns on the part of a health care provider reflect two principles of American health care ethicists: truth-telling to the terminally ill, and patient autonomy.

Within American health care a distinct change in attitude has taken place concerning truth-telling to the terminally ill. Prior to 1960, the predominant practice was to withhold information from the patient, for fear that frank truth would frighten or harm her. (2) Studies indicate that, in 1960, about 90 percent of cancer physicians favored nondisclosure of the diagnosis. But twenty years later, 90 percent favored disclosure of the diagnostic information to patients. (2) *A Patient's Bill of Rights* developed by the American Hospital Association maintains, in general, the right of a patient (or appropriate surrogate) to medical information:

The patient has the right to obtain from his physician complete current information concerning his diagnosis, treatment, and prognosis in terms the patient can be reasonably expected to understand. When it is not medically advisable to give such information to the patient, the information should be made available to an appropriate person in his behalf. (3)

Various concerns have been expressed about a policy of telling the truth to patients who are terminally ill. For one thing, medical diagnoses and prognoses are never 100 percent certain. We can all think of cases in which someone was expected to die but unexpectedly recovered. So why cause a patient distress unnecessarily? Others have questioned the ability of patients who are debilitated by a serious illness to understand the information given to them, and whether patients in fact want bad news communicated to them. Further, there is concern that an announcement of a terminal illness may harm the patient by causing fright or depression, by causing her to cease to struggle against the disease, or even by prompting a cardiac arrest or suicide. (4)

On the other hand, it has been argued that patients often intuitively have a sense of their condition. As Kübler-Ross indicates from her studies with the dying: "When we asked our patients how they had been told, we learned that all the patients know about their terminal illness anyway, whether they were explicitly told or not..." (5) Indeed, patients can be relieved when the issue of their terminal condition is brought out into the open. Proponents of truth-telling also call attention to studies that indicate that a large majority of persons say that they would like to be told of the diagnosis of a serious illness. (4) And it is pointed out that a policy of truth-telling in the case of terminal illness is not equivalent to coldly blurting out medical information. Such a policy can and should be accompanied by "finesse, feeling, warmth, empathy, etc., with regard to how much? when? how?..." (6)

Finally, while concern has been expressed about possible harmful effects on patients of knowing about terminal illness, it is argued that the withholding of information can also have negative consequences:

> ...we are also becoming increasingly aware of all that can befall patients in the course of their illness when information is denied or distorted. Lies place them in a position where they no longer participate in choices concerning their own health, including the choice of whether to be a "patient" in the first place. A terminally ill person who is not informed that his illness is incurable and that he is near death cannot make decisions about the end of his life; about whether or not to enter a hospital, or to have surgery; where and with whom to spend his last days; how to put his affairs in order—these most personal choices cannot be made if he is kept in the dark, or given contradictory hints and clues. (4)

Positively stated, truth-telling to terminally ill patients may allow them to participate in decisions about their medical treatment, to make more satisfying use of the time remaining to them, and to make preparations for death. And this is where there is a connection between truth-telling to the terminally ill and patient autonomy. It is argued that patients should be told the truth about their terminal condition precisely so that they themselves can make choices about and direct what happens at the end of their lives.

To someone imbued with the principles of truth-telling and autonomy (as was the physician caring for Mr. Chang's mother), it might appear that her family is not acting in her best interests. A conflict arises in the case of Mr. Chang's mother precisely because her family is from a culture that brings a different set of beliefs and values to bear in caring for the terminally ill:

> A belief held by many Chinese is that a person is entitled to be treated as a child when ill. Sick adults, like children, deserve "protection." Because a patient is suffering already from the illness, it is unnecessary to make them suffer even more by discussing the reality of the disease. If the patient is gravely ill, the need for protection is perceived as even greater. Among many Asian groups, including the Chinese, to tell someone he or she is dying is not only rude but dangerous. People fear that openly acknowledging an impending death is like casting a death curse upon the person; it will make the person despair and die even sooner. Thus, to engage in discussions of code status or the possibility of hospice care, interventions that can be seen as explicit preparation for death, is courting bad luck.
>
> "Truth telling" also signifies the withdrawing of hope; it tells patients that their physicians have given up on them and they might as well give up, too. Therefore, it would only be an unthinking, callous practitioner who would even consider engaging in an activity with dire consequences. This does not mean that the family and patient necessarily remain unaware of the implications of a grave diagnosis. They many well know and accept the reality of the situation but, at the same time, have a tacit understanding born of cultural expectations about how to behave appropriately in such circumstances—that is, not to acknowledge or discuss it openly. (7)

To this Chinese family, telling Mrs. Chang the truth about her terminal illness is a callous act because it is seen as signifying the loss of all hope and as completely giving up on her. Such truth-telling is considered rude and dangerous. Further, an important value to this family is protecting Mrs. Chang from harm. This value is put into practice by withholding the truth and refraining from any discussions about her impending death. This is a very different mindset from current Western medical practice in which truth-telling is seen positively as something that enables the dying person to have some control over the end of her life.

The attitude of the Chang family is not unique to the Chinese. The practice of not disclosing a terminal illness to a patient is also found among Italians (8), Arabs (1), Ethiopians (9), Mexicans (10), and Koreans (9).

How can health care workers identify when a conflict situation with a resident and his family is due to cultural differences? They can try to learn as much as possible about the cultural beliefs and practices of ethnic groups with whom they have contact. (10) To do this, they might identify one or two individuals from the resident's family or community "who are willing to act as cultural informants." (10) Or they might "consult with other health care practitioners from the same ethnic group" as the resident. (10) Or they might call on the resources of local colleges and universities. (10)

How can health care workers resolve conflicts due to cultural differences? Health care workers need to be flexible: they need to show respect for beliefs and practices different from their own, and they need to be willing to compromise. (10) For example, in the case of Mr.Chang and his mother an accommodation might be achieved between American and Chinese values by the physician asking Mrs. Chang if she has any questions about her condition or treatment, and by assuring Mr. Chang that his mother will not be told any more than she wishes to know. (10) Ethically, these accommodations to persons of different cultures respect their right to self-determination and autonomy. (10)

Further Examples of Cultural Diversity

In the above case, Dr. Marilyn Scott feels that Mr. Chang is being unfair to his mother in not allowing her to be informed of her terminal condition for the reason that "it's her life and it should be up to her to decide what treatments she does and does not want." This statement indicates how truth-telling to the terminally ill is related to the value of individual autonomy. An argument given in favor of truth-telling is that knowledge of a terminal condition will empower individuals to make choices about and direct what happens at the end of their lives.

As evident throughout this book, autonomy is a prominent value in contemporary health care ethics. In the context of end-of-life decision making, several authors have described the emphasis on autonomy in this way:

> Traditionally, bioethics theory and practice have relied heavily on the Western philosophical principle of respect for persons to justify a model of end-of-life decision making that is focused on the rights and wishes of the individual patient. An important goal of bioethics innovations—such as advance care directives and open disclosure of prognosis—is to promote control of medical decision making at the end of life by an autonomous, fully informed patient.

> In the United States, the "ideal" patient is a self-governing individual who is future oriented and willing to engage in frank discussions about difficult medical topics, including planning for his or her own death. (11)

However, "some have argued that this preoccupation with individual rights to the exclusion of other values," such as family integrity and physician responsibility, "may reflect a cultural bias on the part of the Western medical and bioethics communities." (9) It has been suggested that "the notion of an informed active decision maker may not be a universally held ideal of the good patient but rather, a very specific set of values based on a particular Western philosophical tradition." (11)

For example, one study discovered that Korean Americans (28 percent) and Mexican Americans (41 percent) were less likely than African Americans (60 percent) and European Americans (65 percent) to believe that the patient should be the one to make decisions about the use of life-supporting technology. (9) The investigators found that

> The decision-making style exhibited by most of the Mexican-American and Korean-American subjects in our study might best be described as family centered. Although the patient autonomy model does not exclude family involvement, in this family-centered model, it is the sole responsibility of the family to hear bad news about the patient's diagnosis and prognosis and to make the difficult decisions about life support. (9)

Similarly, others have noted that "in many Asian societies, ideas about 'selfhood' vary from the western ideal of an autonomous individual." (12) Concomitantly, a "sociocentric or relational sense of self often leads to decision-making styles at odds with western bioethics ideals." (12)

Cultural differences have also become apparent in attitudes about using life-sustaining treatments. Studies indicate "European-Americans are more likely than other ethnic populations to complete a living will or durable power of attorney." (11) Further, African-Americans are "more likely than Anglos to agree to initiate life support," and they are also "more likely to disagree with stopping life support." (11) Similarly, a study conducted in Miami found that significantly more Hispanic patients "wanted their doctors to keep them alive regardless of how ill they were, while more...whites agreed to stop life-prolonging treatment under some circumstances." (11)

Cultural differences in approaches to health care extend beyond the realm of end-of-life care. For example, it is commonplace in the United States to have individuals sign a written consent form for a variety of diagnostic tests and medical procedures. However, an Arab who has verbally agreed to a test or procedure may become irate when subsequently asked to sign a written consent form and may refuse to do so. (1) This is because Arabs regard a verbal agreement as "binding and equal to their written agreement." (1) To press them further for a written agreement "only suggests mistrust of their verbal contract" and challenges their personal honor. (1)

What does this cultural diversity mean for ethics and the validity of ethical judgments and practices? Can we ever say for sure that anything is ethically right or wrong?

Ethical Relativism vs. Ethical Absolutism

Multiculturalism in health care raises the question of *ethical absolutism* versus *ethical relativism*. Ethical absolutists maintain that there is one, objectively true set of ethical standards and values that holds for everyone everywhere. An ethical relativist, on the other hand, denies this and maintains that what is in fact right and wrong varies among different cultures and groups. So, for example, an ethical relativist might maintain that polygamy (the practice of having more than one wife at the same time) is ethically wrong in one country but ethically right in another. The ethical relativist does *not* maintain merely that people in the two countries may *think* polygamy is wrong (or right), but that polygamy is *in fact* wrong in one country but right in another.

That different cultural groups do in fact consider different things to be ethically right and wrong is often presented as evidence in favor of ethical relativism. For example, Americans favor telling the complete and absolute truth about terminal illness to a patient whereas this is considered the wrong thing to do by Chinese, Koreans, Arabs, Ethiopians, Italians, and Mexicans. But does this really mean there is no shared morality among all human beings?

Those favoring ethical absolutism argue that different cultures and groups may share the same basic ethical principles and values but may put these principles and values into practice in different ways because of different circumstances or a different set of factual beliefs. For example, in the aforementioned case of giving consent to a medical procedure, the consent itself is really not at issue. The question concerns the way giving consent is practiced. Americans emphasize written consent whereas Arabs place a high value on verbal consent. In the case of Mr. Chang and his mother we learn that Chinese place a high priority on protecting patients from harm. American health care ethicists adhere to the principle of nonmaleficence, recognizing an obligation of health care workers to prevent harm from coming to patients and residents. Thus the same basic value is held in the two cultures, and the dispute arises over the consequences believed to follow from truth-telling in the case of terminal illness. Chinese see truth-telling as harming a patient by causing her to lose hope and thus bringing on an earlier death. Americans, on the other hand, have questioned whether these bad effects really come about for most dying persons and see harm coming from withholding the truth about terminal illness. Thus, if Chinese and Americans could be brought to agree on the consequences of truth-telling in the case of terminal illness, they might well agree ethically on whether this should be done.

FOR GROUP DISCUSSION

1. What ethnic and racial groups are present in your geographical area? How much do you know about their beliefs and practices regarding the provision of health care? Where or from whom can you find out more information?

2. Considering your own role in health care, have you ever been faced with a dilemma or conflict situation stemming from a difference of culture? When you analyze the situation, can you see any common, underlying values shared by those involved in the situation? How was the situation resolved? How do you think it should have been resolved?

3. The federal Patient Self-Determination Act (PSDA) requires health care facilities to provide information to patients and residents about advance directives at the time of admission. If you are connected with a long-term care facility, what provisions have been made by your facility for explaining advance

directives to people of diverse cultures who may seek admission to the facility? Do you think these provisions are adequate?

4. As previously mentioned, studies indicate that African-Americans and Hispanic-Americans are less likely to be willing to stop life-sustaining treatments than white Americans. Can you speculate about what might account for this difference in attitude ?

NOTES

1. Afaf Ibrahim Meleis & Albert R. Jonsen, "Ethical Crises and Cultural Differences," *The Western Journal of Medicine* 138/6 (June 1983): 889-93.
2. Howard Brody, "The Physician/Patient Relationship" in Robert M. Veatch (ed.), *Medical Ethics* (Boston: Jones and Bartlett, 1989).
3. Special Committee on Biomedical Ethics of the American Hospital Association, *Values in Conflict Resolving Ethical Issues in Hospital Care* (Chicago: American Hospital Association, 1985).
4. Sissela Bok, "Lies to the Sick and Dying" in *Lying: Moral Choice in Public and Private Life* (New York: Pantheon, 1978).
5. Elisabeth Kübler-Ross, *On Death and Dying* (New York: Macmillan, 1969).
6. Orville N. Griese, *Catholic Identity in Health Care: Principles and Practice* (Braintree: MA: Pope John Center, 1987).
7. Jessica H. Muller & Brian Desmond, "Ethical Dilemmas in a Cross-cultural Context A Chinese Example," *The Western Journal of Medicine* 157/3 (Sept. 1992): 323-7.
8. Antonella Surbone, "Letter from Italy Truth Telling to the Patient," *Journal of the American Medical Association* 268/13 (Oct. 7, 1992): 1661-2.
9. Leslie J. Blackhall, Sheila T. Murphy, Gelya Frank, Vicki Michel, and Stanley Azen, "Ethnicity and Attitudes Toward Patient Autonomy," *Journal of the American Medical Association* 274/10 (Sept. 13, 1995): 820-5.
10. Robert D. Orr, Patricia A. Marshall & Jamie Osborn, "Cross-cultural Considerations in Clinical Ethics Consultations," *Archives of Family Medicine* 4 (Feb. 1995): 159-64.
11. Patricia A. Marshall, Barbara A. Koenig, Donelle M. Barnes, and Anne J. Davis, "Multiculturalism, Bioethics, and End-of-Life Care: Case Narratives of Latino Cancer Patients" in John F. Monagle and David C. Thomasma (eds.), *Health Care Ethics: Critical Issues for the 21st Century* (Gaithersburg, MD: Aspen, 1998).
12. Barbara A.Koenig and Jan Gates-Williams, "Understanding Cultural Difference in Caring for Dying Patients," *Western Journal of Medicine* 163/3 (Sept. 1995): 244-9.

FOR FURTHER STUDY

• Darryl Wieland, Donna Benton, B. Josea Kramer, Grace D. Dawson (eds.), *Cultural Diversity and Geriatric Care Challenges to the Health Professions* (New York: Haworth, 1994). This book contains papers presented at a conference held in August 1993, in Los Angeles.

- Robert M. Veatch (ed.), *Cross-Cultural Perspectives in Medical Ethics: Readings* (Boston: Jones and Bartlett, 1989), Chapter 3 "Medical Ethical Theories Outside the Anglo-American West."

- *Journal of Transcultural Nursing.* 1990 - present. Sage Publications, Inc. (2455 Teller Rd. Thousand Oaks, CA 91320-2218) Tel. 805-499-0721. info@sagepub.com

- Vernellia R. Randall, "Ethnic Americans, Long-Term Health Care Providers, and the Patient Self-Determination Act" in Marshall B. Kapp (ed.), *Patient Self-Determination in Long-Term Care Implementing the PSDA in Medical Decisions* (New York: Springer, 1994).

- Ake Hultkrantz, *Shamanic Healing and Ritualistic Drama Health and Medicine in the Native North American Religious Traditions* (New York: Crossroad, 1997).

- Earle H. Waugh, *Islamic Tradition Religious Beliefs and Healthcare Decisions* (Chicago: Park Ridge Center, 1999).

- Fazlur Rahman, *Health and Medicine in the Islamic Tradition* (New York: Crossroad, 1987).

- Paul D. Numrich, *Buddhist Tradition Religious Beliefs and Healthcare Decisions* (Chicago: Park Ridge Center, 2001).

Part Four

Special Topics

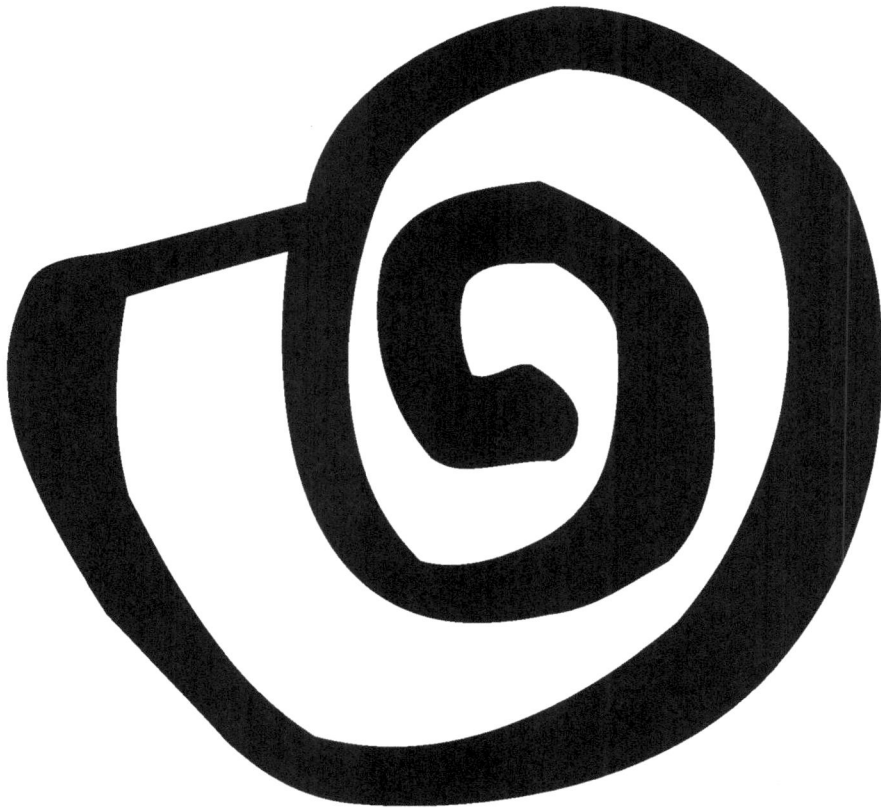

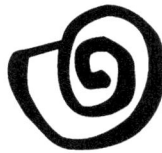

Chapter 18

Pain Management

The issue of pain and pain control has surfaced in the current debate over euthanasia and assisted suicide. Surveys show that "as many as two-thirds of Americans support some form of medically assisted death." (1) However, research also shows that "when people are presented with another option—compassionate hospice care and, especially, good pain control for the dying—only 13 percent say they would still choose physician-assisted suicide." (1)

Pain at the end of life is not uncommon. It occurs "in up to 90% of cancer patients, 80% of AIDS patients in the terminal phase, and 60% of patients dying of end-stage organ failure." (2) But good pain management is important not just at the end of life. A particular challenge in the long-term care setting is dealing with the chronic pain of residents. It has been estimated that 45 percent to 85 percent of nursing home residents suffer from chronic pain. (3) Further, "there is accumulating evidence that the problem of pain undertreatment, well documented in acute care and oncology populations, is also a serious concern for the elderly and for residents of long-term care, in particular." (4)

The Joint Commission on Accreditation of Healthcare Organizations (JCAHO) has introduced pain management into its standards for long-term care. (5) Affirming that "The resident has a right to appropriate assessment and management of pain" [RI.2.6], the standards recommend that a resident's pain and the current treatment for it be assessed at the time of admission [PE.2.1.10] and be regularly reassessed thereafter [Intent of RI.2.6], that health care workers be educated in pain assessment and management [Intent of RI.2.6], and also that residents and family members be educated about their roles in managing pain [Intent of RI.2.6]. A long-term care facility should communicate to residents and their families that pain management is an important part of care [Intent of RI.2.6], and residents should be aware of when and how to seek help for pain management in conjunction with their treatments [Intent of PF.3.5].

This chapter covers:
• *the ethical imperative of health care workers to provide good pain management;*
• *barriers to good pain management;*
• *specific ethical issues involved with pain management;*
• *pain management and impairment of mental functioning.*

CASE STUDIES

Marjorie Burke has recently assumed the position of director of nursing (DON) at the Cedar Grove Retirement Community, a multi-level facility ranging from assisted living apartments to a skilled nursing unit. Shortly after beginning work, she encounters two disturbing situations.

The first case involves Ruth and Tom Jackson. Ruth and Tom have been married for over forty years. Six years ago they moved into an apartment in the assisted living unit. Three years ago Ruth was found to have stomach and colon cancer. Since that time she has undergone aggressive chemotherapy treatment. However, it was recently discovered that the cancer has spread to Ruth's pancreas.

Two weeks ago Ruth was placed in the skilled nursing unit. Rather than going to a hospital, she wanted to stay at Cedar Grove because that is "her home." Her weight is down to 95 pounds, and friends who come to see her remark how much she has "aged." Her pain is constant. Although Ruth is receiving pain medication once every four hours, it doesn't seem strong enough to really help her.

Tom spent last night at his wife's side. Her pain and discomfort were so severe that she wasn't able to sleep. She tried praying but could not concentrate because of the pain. It was even difficult for her husband to converse with her. All he could do was sit and hold her hand while she twisted and turned in bed. Occasionally Ruth would scream that she wished God would take her.

Late the next evening, Tom is still keeping vigil at his wife's bedside. When Ruth finally falls asleep, Tom kisses her for the last time, takes a pillow, and smothers her.

Tom readily admits to what he did, and he may face criminal charges for trying to relieve his wife's suffering. The entire Cedar Grove staff is shaken by this incident. When Marjorie sees the oncologist who has been in charge of Ruth's case, she asks him if more couldn't have been done to relieve Ruth's pain. Marjorie wonders whether Ruth's caregivers are not the ones ultimately responsible for this tragedy.

*   *   *

Mildred Wolfe, 80, suffers from osteoporosis and arthritis. Before she entered the Cedar Grove Retirement Community, her physician prescribed medication for her condition, but Mildred had to stop taking it because it caused stomach bleeding. At present, Mildred relies on over the counter arthritis medication, which really doesn't help her all that much. The incident with stomach bleeding has left her terribly afraid to "try anything stronger" from a doctor.

Mildred not only has difficulty walking, but even in getting up from a chair. Sometimes she doesn't want to get dressed at all because her arms hurt so much when she lifts them to put on her clothes. She is obviously depressed, and she only eats one meal a day despite the patient coaxing of staff.

Marjorie has always considered herself to be a patient advocate. For this reason, she decides to raise the issue of pain management at the next care conference for Mildred.

Pain Management: The Ethical Imperative

Pain is much more than the experience of an unpleasant sensation. It can affect a person physically, mentally, emotionally, socially, and spiritually. (6) It can negatively impact a person's whole life. This is evident in the case of Mildred Wolfe. Pain can be so overwhelming that it is all someone can think about. It can even destroy a person's will to live. (7)

> Unrelieved pain has a number of adverse physiological and psychological consequences, including impaired gastrointestinal and pulmonary function, impaired immune response, insomnia, loss of appetite, inability to walk or move about, anxiety and depression, loss of enjoyment of life, inability to maintain close relationships, feelings of hopelessness and helplessness, and even requests for physician-assisted suicide. (8)

In Cardinal Bernardin's book *The Gift of Peace* we have a firsthand report of the deleterious effects of experiencing pain:

> ...I experienced the discomforts one normally encounters after going through extensive surgery. I wanted to pray, but the physical discomfort was overwhelming. I remember saying to the friends who visited me, "Pray while you're well, because if you wait until you're sick you might not be able to do it." They looked at me, astonished. I said, "I'm in so much discomfort that I can't focus on prayer. My faith is still present. There is nothing wrong with my faith, I'm just too preoccupied with the pain...." (9)

One of the central values of health care ethics is *beneficence*. This is the moral obligation of health care workers to promote the health and well being of patients. Because of the wide range of harmful effects that pain can have, beneficence mandates that health care workers provide good pain management for individuals under their care. (10)

From another perspective, health care workers have an obligation to affirm the *values of compassion and humanity* by mitigating pain and suffering. (11) Concomitantly, "they have a responsibility to be technically competent in palliation and pain relief and to provide adequate symptom control." (11)

Moreover, as seen in the case of Ruth Jackson, severe uncontrolled pain can lead to a desire for euthanasia or assisted suicide. For those who find these practices to be ethically objectionable, this consequence of unrelieved pain provides additional reason for asserting an ethical imperative for good pain management.

Challenges in Providing Pain Management

Many different factors are barriers to good pain management.

One factor is a lack of training of health care workers in good pain management techniques. Many health care workers simply do not know what is available for pain management and how to use it effectively. (1,11) This certainly seems to be true in both of the cases described above. Due to her cancer Ruth Jackson is described as suffering intense pain but "studies indicate that as many as 95 percent" of cancer patients "can get good pain relief if skilled practitioners administer the right medications in the right ways." (1) In the second case of Mildred Wolfe, her chronic unrelieved and debilitating pain should long ago have triggered a review of her treatment regimen by nursing home staff and by her physician. Are there newer pain medications that she could tolerate? Could she benefit from the use of topical agents? Or from nondrug therapies like stretching and strengthening exercises? (3)

In achieving better pain management in the long-term care setting, it is important to focus attention on certified nursing assistants (CNAs) as the staff members with the most direct contact with residents. CNAs need to know what to observe and to report, and what they can do to comfort residents in pain. Some facilities have also trained housekeeping and dietary staff on what to observe and report to the nursing staff so that nurses can respond promptly even to nonverbal evidence of pain. (4)

Another significant factor, affecting both health care workers and residents, is fear of the person becoming *addicted* to the pain medication. (2, 4, 7, 10, 11, 12, 13) Could this be a reason why Ruth Jackson was not given medication in doses sufficient to control her pain while she was in the nursing home?

Actually, the fear of addiction is unwarranted. First, addiction rarely occurs in a health care setting. One estimate is that "less than 0.1% of patients develop addiction." (7; see also 14) Second, it is possible for a patient to take strong opioids for a length of time to control pain, and then to get off the drug. (15) Further, a distinction can be made between *addiction* and *drug dependence*. In the case of drug dependency, the drug has a medical value for the person taking it. The dependency is a physical, rather than a psychological, problem. Withdrawal symptoms will occur if the drug is taken away suddenly, so that the drug needs to be taken away gradually, over a period of time. Addiction, on the other hand, is a psychological problem. The drug has no medical value for the person taking it, but the individual desires it and is driven to obtain it. (11, 15) If Ruth Jackson had been given pain medication in doses sufficient to control her severe pain, she would undoubtedly have become physically dependent on it, but this does not mean that she should be considered an "addict." Moreover, in the case of someone who is dying, like Ruth Jackson, the pain medication need never be stopped to cause withdrawal symptoms. (11)

Cultural factors may also hinder good pain management. In the minds of some people the term "narcotic" (that is, opioid) automatically evokes an image of street drugs. (15) We are all familiar with the slogan, "Just say no to drugs." (14) Unfortunately, the stigma attached to opioids may carry over into the health care setting, where such drugs have perfectly legitimate uses. (16)

There are also reasons why some people may not want to say that they are in pain. Our society has the idea that "real men can take it" and don't need pain relief. (15) Some may fear that others will judge them "as weak, as wimps" if they express being in pain. (10) And "good" patients just don't complain to the staff taking care of them. (17, 18)

Some "believe that continuous and increasing pain indicates a progression of their disease" and, for this reason, "they become reluctant to admit any increase in pain either to themselves or to their caregivers." (7; see also13) This could also be a factor in the case of Mildred Wolfe. Side effects of pain medication, such as drowsiness, constipation, and mental confusion, may also make individuals unwilling to take pain medication. (14)

In addition to all of these factors, there are challenges to providing good pain management unique to the long-term care setting. For example, it may be more difficult to assess pain in long-term care residents because of visual and hearing impairments, cognitive impairments, multiple diagnoses, multiple pain sites, multiple medications, and the cultural myth that pain is a normal part of aging. (19, 20) Moreover, "there are physician, nursing, institutional and regulatory barriers that impede pain management" in the long-term care setting "above and beyond the already familiar barriers to pain management in hospitalized patients." (21)

> First, as a heavily regulated industry, especially concerning the use of psychoactive medication, LTCF nurses and physicians are hesitant to use scheduled analgesics for chronic pain out of fear of regulatory scrutiny by state or federal surveyors. Second, most pain experienced by LTCF residents is non-malignant and to date there has been little acceptance by physicians of routinely scheduled opioid therapy for chronic non-malignant pain, although increasing evidence points to the relative safety and efficacy of opioids for this indication. Third, physician involvement in the day-to-day care of LTCF residents is far less than for hospitalized patients. Contact typically occurs only once every 30 days. Fourth, the bulk of actual patient contact in the LTCF is via certified nursing assistants, who have little to no training in pain assessment. (21)

For these reasons, the Medical College of Wisconsin Palliative Care Program began a model project in 1996. (20, 21) Working with eighty-seven long-term care facilities in Eastern Wisconsin, the project included use of "individualized pain assessment tools for cognitively impaired and unimpaired patients, use of a standardized pain scale and a pain flow sheet document, specific pain protocols and policies, an interdisciplinary pain program and a patient satisfaction survey program." (20) Other features of the project included "a quality improvement process, resident and family pain education, and new staff orientation for all nursing, rehabilitation and support staff." (20) This project was the first of its kind in the United States and is drawing national interest. (20)

Ethical Issues in Pain Management

The traditional ethical question about pain management has concerned the use of pain medications that may hasten death. For example, morphine may depress respiration and, in this way, have a secondary effect of hastening the sick person's death. This secondary effect has made some health care workers hesitant about administering such pain medications. They fear they are engaging in an act of euthanasia. These concerns might well arise in a case like that of Ruth Jackson, where high doses of opioids would likely be needed to control her severe cancer pain.

Traditionally, the answer has been given that it is indeed morally permissible to use medications to relieve pain that may have a side effect of hastening the time of death. This position has been justified using the ethical *principle of double effect*. (1, 2) This principle applies to situations in which a single action will have two different consequences. One of the consequences is perfectly good and is what is intended. The second consequence, however, is bad and is not really wanted, but it comes along as a side effect of the action. The principle of double effect says that it is morally permissible to take an action with such double consequences. More exactly, the principle of double effect can be stated as follows:

> This doctrine, which is designed to provide moral guidance for an action that could have at least one bad and one good effect, holds that such an action is permissible if it satisfies these four conditions: (1) The act itself must be morally good or neutral (for example, administering a pain-killer); (2) only the good consequences of the action must be intended (relief of the patient's suffering); (3) the good effect must not be produced by means of the evil effect (the relief of suffering must not be produced by the patient's death); (4) there must be some weighty reason for permitting the evil (the relief of great suffering, which can only be achieved through a high risk of death). (22)

Intent is critical in using the principle of double effect. It must be pain relief, not the sick person's death, which is intended in administering the medication. But how does one know someone's intent in administering pain medication? This is one way: if a certain dosage level of the pain medication relieves the person's pain, the level will not be deliberately increased to risk depression of respiration (and death). This indicates that the intent is indeed to relieve pain.

Fortunately, this ethical concern about pain medication is becoming outdated. First of all, "there is some evidence that administering narcotic agents in amounts sufficient to provide adequate pain relief may extend, rather than shorten, life." (11) This is so because "patients without pain are more likely to accept a greater degree of nourishment, to be more active and less depressed, and to be more open to other treatment possibilities," and, "as a result, they may live longer." (11) Second, more is now known about how to administer pain medication in a way that avoids depression of respiration:

> Health care professionals who are accustomed to giving one to two milligrams of morphine in the emergency room or coronary care unit for the relief of moderate acute pain need to know that some patients may need, and can tolerate, 1,000 milligrams or more of morphine per hour, as in intravenous infusion, to control the ferocious pain of some cancers. Such doses are not reached overnight but infusions are judiciously titrated upwards in measured increments until pain is contained. In this way respiratory distress does not occur, since unrelieved pain acts as a physiological antagonist to the respiratory depressant effect of the opiate drug. (10)

Finally, it is now recognized that respiratory depression and arrest is a normal part of the dying process, and we need to be careful not to falsely see it as caused by pain medication:

However, current medical research raises questions about the need to apply the principle of double effect to pain management. As the chair of the Wisconsin Cancer Pain Initiative stated in correspondence to the Council of Ethical and Judicial Affairs of the American Medical Association, "Death from respiratory depression is exceedingly rare in patients with cancer who chronically receive opioid analgesics for pain. As a person nears death, there is deterioration in respiratory function. However, these respiratory changes should not be confused with the effects of opioids. (23)

In sum, there is no reason to withhold adequate doses of pain medication from persons who are dying for fear of hastening their death.

At the institutional level, there is an often-unrecognized ethical issue about pain management. In order to achieve good pain management, a facility must be willing to make a substantial commitment of its resources (as described, for example, in the Medical College of Wisconsin's model project) to ensure that the needs of each of its residents is met. In other words, pain management must be made an institutional priority. Ethically, this kind of commitment is grounded in the principle of distributive justice, which concerns fairness in the distribution of benefits and resources and the treatment of individuals according to their need. (23)

Pain Management and the Impairment of Mental Functioning

On some occasions the administration of medication adequate to relieve severe pain may impair the person's mental functioning, causing confusion, reducing decision-making capacity, or even reducing or suppressing consciousness. In respect for the individual's autonomy, the resident should be consulted when pain medication is likely to have these effects. The resident should have the opportunity to decide what level of pain, if any, she is prepared to tolerate as a trade-off for mental clarity. (11) The resident may want to remain mentally alert for some period in order to take care of unfinished business matters, visit with family members and friends, or prepare spiritually for death.

It is estimated that over 90 percent of pain can be relieved, and usually by means of drugs. (2, 10) However, this leaves a residue of unrelieved pain. In these cases, some find euthanasia or assisted suicide attractive as a way of relieving the suffering of persons who are already dying. (24) An alternative choice in cases of unrelievable pain experienced by the dying is sedation to the point of unconsciousness on a continuing basis:

If the only troubling issue that arises...is that of having to accept unconsciousness in order to avoid severe pain, this is a morally acceptable course. ...It may be that a brief life of nearly continuous sedation is not of great merit, even though it is better than any other life that can be made available. ...However, continuous sedation achieves a humane and compassionate period of dying for patient, caregivers, and family without precipitating the very serious concerns about "slippery slopes" that arise with acceptance of direct killing. Therefore, sedation is the best policy in the unusual instance of pain so severe that it cannot be relieved while still keeping the patient awake. (25)

Again, this course of action should be discussed with and agreed to by the resident out of respect for his autonomy. (25)

FOR GROUP DISCUSSION

1. Can you remember an instance in which you experienced significant pain? How did it affect your attitudes and your ability to function? Were you satisfied with the pain relief measures you received?

2. This chapter has discussed various misconceptions, fears, attitudes, and ethical concerns that can affect pain management. Have you encountered any of these within your own family? Among residents to whom you have provided care? Among co-workers?

3. It has been suggested that pain management should be included in a facility's mission statement, resident bill of rights, and other important documents. (4) Review significant documents from your facility. Is pain management mentioned anywhere? In what documents do you think it would be appropriate to include a commitment to good pain management?

4. In the context of your own particular job or role in health care, how do you think you can promote good pain management?

NOTES

1. Phebe Saunders Haugen, "Pain Relief Legal Aspects of Pain Relief for the Dying," *Minnesota Medicine* 80 (Nov. 1997): 15-18.
2. Thomas E. Elliott, "Pain Control at the End of Life," *Minnesota Medicine* 80 (Nov. 1997): 27-32.
3. C. Michael Stein, Marie R. Griffin, Jo A. Taylor et al., " An educational program for nursing home patients and staff to reduce use of non-steroidal anti-inflammatory drugs among nursing home residents: A randomized controlled trial," *Medical Care* 39 (May 2001): 436-45.
4. Judith A. Spross, "Harnessing Power and Passion: Lessons from Pain Management Leaders and Literature," *Innovations in End-of-Life Care* 3/1 (2001). http://www.edc.org/last acts
5. Joint Commission on Accreditation of Healthcare Organizations, 2002-2003 *Standards for Long Term Care* (Oakbrook Terrace, IL: Joint Commission Resources, 2002).
6. Joanne Lynn and Joan Harrold, *Handbook for Mortals Guidance for People Facing Serious Illness* (New York: Oxford University Press, 1999).
7. Edwin L. Lisson, "Ethical Issues in Pain Management," *Seminars in Oncology Nursing* 5/2 (May 1989): 114-19.
8. June L. Dahl, Patricia Berry, Karen M. Stevenson, Debra B. Gordon, Sandra Ward, "Institutionalizing Pain Management: Making Pain Assessment and Treatment an Integral Part of the Nation's Healthcare System," *American Pain Society* (APS) Bulletin 8/4 (July/August 1998). http://www.ampainsoc.org/pub/bulletin

9. Joseph Cardinal Bernardin, *The Gift of Peace* (Chicago: Loyola Press, 1997).

10. Catholic Health Association of the United States, *Care of the Dying* (St. Louis: Catholic Health Association of the United States, 1993).

11. Hastings Center, *Guidelines on the Termination of Life-Sustaining Treatment and the Care of the Dying* (Briarcliff Manor, NY: The Hastings Center, 1987).

12. American Geriatrics Society, *Proposed Guidelines for the Management of Chronic Nonmalignant Pain in the Elderly Long-Term Care Resident: The Relief Paradigm.* http://www.macmcm.com/ascp/ascp98-agsgmp.htm

13. L. Jean Dunegan, "The Ethics of Pain Management," *Annals of Long Term Care* 8/11 (2000): 23-6.

14. Chia-chin Lin, "Enhancing Management of Cancer Pain: Contribution of the Internal Working Model," *Cancer Nursing* 21/2 (1998): 90-6.

15. *Quality of Mercy A Case for Better Pain Management*, a video produced by Richard J. Adler (New York: Filmakers Library).

16. Russell K. Portenoy et al., "Pain Management and Chemical Dependency," *Journal of the American Medical Association* 278/7 (August 20, 1997): 592-3.

17. Gail C. Davis, "Nursing's Role in Pain Management Across the Health Care Continuum," *Nursing Outlook* (Jan./Feb. 1998): 19-23.

18. Alice M. Wagner et al., "Pain Prevalence and Pain Treatments for Residents in Oregon Nursing Homes, " *Geriatric Nursing* 18/6 (Nov./Dec. 1997): 268-72.

19. S.L. Sodickson, "Changing Pain Management Practice at Franciscan Woods: An Interview with Mary Arata," *Innovations in End-of-Life Care* 3/1 (2001). http://www.edc.org/lastacts

20. Medical College of Wisconsin, News Release "Medical College Team Leads Effort to Improve Pain Management in Long-Term Care Facilities," December 4, 1999. http://www.mcw.edu/news/html/news_release_991204.html

21. David E. Weissman, Julie Griffie, Sandra Muchka, Sandra Matson, "Improving Pain Management in Long-Term Care Facilities," *Innovations in End-of-Life Care* 3/1 (2001). http://www.edc.org/lastacts

22. President's Commission for the Study of Ethical Problems in Medicine and Biomedical and Behavioral Research, *Deciding to Forego Life-Sustaining Treatment* (1983; reprint New York: Concern for Dying).

23. Task Force on Pain Management of the Catholic Health Association, "Pain Management," *Health Progress* (Jan.-Feb. 1993): 30-40.

24. See, for example, Lonny Shavelson, *A Chosen Death The Dying Confront Assisted Suicide* (New York: Simon & Schuster, 1995).

25. Joanne Lynn, "Morpheus or Death: The Case of Nicholas Miklovick" in Cynthia B. Cohen (ed.), *Casebook on the Termination of Life-Sustaining Treatment and the Care of the Dying* (Bloomington, IN: Indiana University Press, 1988).

FOR FURTHER STUDY

• J. Griffie, S. Matson, S. Muchka, D.E. Weissman, *Improving Pain Management in Long-Term Care Settings: A Resource Guide for Institutional Change* (Milwaukee: Medical College of Wisconsin, 1998).

• J. Griffie, D.E. Weissman, *Nursing Staff Education Resource Manual: A Six Session Inservice Education Program in Pain Management for Long-Term Care Faciltie*s (Milwaukee: Medical College of Wisconsin, 2000).

- American Medical Directors Association, *Clinical Practice Guideline: Chronic Pain Managment in the Long-Term Care Setting* (Columbia, MD: American Medical Directors Association, 1999).

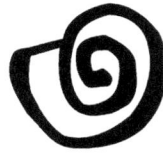

Chapter 19

Research and Experimentation Involving Human Subjects

The Nuremberg trials following World War II brought to light medical research and experimentation conducted by the Nazis that was abusive of human subjects. These abuses were prevalent in the concentration camps. At Dachau, for example, "healthy inmates were injected with extracts from the mucous glands of mosquitoes to produce malaria" and then various drugs were "used to determine their relative effectiveness." (1) At Buchenwald "various kinds of poisons were secretly administered to a number of inmates to test their efficacy." (1) At Ravensbrueck people were deliberately cut and their wounds infected with bacteria in order to test the efficacy of the drug sulfanilamide. (1)

Unfortunately, medical experiments abusive of human beings were not limited to Nazi Germany. Questionable research projects have also been conducted within the United States. A prime example is the Tuskegee Syphilis Study conducted under the auspices of the U.S. Department of Public Health:

> From 1932 to 1970, a large but undetermined number of black males suffering from the later stages of syphilis were examined at regular intervals to determine the course their disease was taking. The men in the study were poor and uneducated... they were given either no treatment or inadequate treatment, and at least forty of them died as a result of factors connected with their disease... It was known when the study began that those with untreated syphilis have a higher death rate than those whose condition is treated, and although the study was started before the advent of penicillin (which is highly effective against syphilis), other drugs were available but were not used in ways to produce the best results. When penicillin became generally available, it still was not used. (1)

This is not an isolated incident. From the 1940s to the 1960s chemical testing involving mescaline and LSD was conducted by the American military and intelligence agencies. Experiments took place without the knowledge of the subjects and sometimes resulted in death. (2) Also controversial were the Willowbrook hepatitis experiments, which involved mentally retarded children in a state institution as research subjects. (1)

Such abusive practices have led to the formulation of codes of research ethics such as the *Nuremberg Code* (3) and the *Declaration of Helsinki* of the World Medical Association (4). Within the United States health care facilities and research institutes have established institutional review boards (IRBs) to review and approve proposed research projects as a condition for receiving funding from the U.S. Department of Health and Human Services. (2)

This chapter covers:
- *general norms and specific criteria used to evaluate proposed research projects;*
- *ethical principles underlying these norms and criteria;*
- *the application of these norms and principles within a long-term care setting.*

CASE STUDY

Marilyn Stewart provides occupational therapy services at Sun Valley Care Center. When she makes her visit this week, the administrator calls Marilyn into his office. He tells her that researchers at the state university medical school are conducting a study of a new blood pressure medication using the residents of Sun Valley. This new medication is expected to have fewer of the unpleasant side effects many older persons experience with the currently standard medications. However, the administrator points out that "you can never be sure exactly what to expect with medication that is still being tested." He asks Marilyn to watch for unusual symptoms or behavior on the part of residents—which may be a function of the medication—and to alert a nurse on duty about it.

Marilyn notices that the administrator seems quite proud that his facility was chosen by researchers at the state university's medical school to participate in this study. However, she wonders how much the residents themselves understand about the research project in which they are the experimental subjects. Some of the residents are hard of hearing and have poor eyesight. Some suffer from memory loss. Some suffer from dementia, in varying degrees. What kind of explanation of the research study was given to the residents? And how much of the explanation did they in fact understand? Who made the decision that the residents should participate in this research project? Marilyn wonders if the residents of whom she has grown so fond are simply being used as "guinea pigs."

Norms and Criteria for Evaluating Proposed Research Projects

Before this new blood pressure medication could be administered to the residents of Sun Valley Care Center, the researchers would have been required to submit a proposal to the Institutional Review Board (IRB) at the university's medical school to conduct this study. The members of the IRB would review their research protocol to ensure proper protection for the human subjects to be used in the research project. In their review, the members of the IRB might use something like the following worksheet.

IRB Worksheet

...(R)esearch will be founded on the four basic principles for human conduct: beneficence (doing good), nonmaleficence (not harming), respecting persons and justice. The proposal is reviewed using six ethical norms for research involving human subjects founded on these principles. The criteria listed are conditions each of which must be satisfied for a project to be ethically legitimate...

1) **Good research design**
   1.1 Based on a thorough knowledge of the scientific literature.
   1.2 Designed and based on results of experimentation at the pre-human level, if available.
   1.3 Conforms to generally accepted scientific principles.
   1.4 Expected to yield fruitful results for the good of society, unprocurable by other methods or means of study.
   1.5 Conducted so as to avoid all unnecessary physical and mental suffering and injury.
   1.6 Importance of the objective is in proportion to the inherent risk to the subject.
   1.7 Confidentiality: Every precaution is taken to respect the privacy of the subject and to minimize the impact of the study on the subject's physical and mental integrity and on the personality of the subject. In publication of the results, the doctor is obliged to preserve the accuracy of the results.

2) **Balance of harm and benefit**
   2.1 Degree of risk to be taken does not exceed that determined by the humanitarian importance of the problem to be solved by the experiment.
   2.2 Preceded by careful assessment of predictable risks in comparison with foreseeable benefits to the subject or to others.
   2.3 Concern for the interests of the subject always prevails over the interest of science and society.

3) **Competence of the investigator(s)**
   3.1 Investigator (or investigative team) has adequate training and skill to accomplish the purposes of the research.
   3.2 Supervision by a clinically competent medical person.
   3.3 A high degree of professionalism with evidence of responsibility for the human subject.

4) Informed Consent

4.1 Voluntary consent of the human subject is absolutely essential.

4.2 Person involved has legal capacity to give consent (OR if the person is legally incompetent, guardian consents; OR if a minor, responsible relative consents in addition to minor consent).

4.3 Person or proxy acknowledges sufficient knowledge and comprehension of the elements of the research project (aims, methods, anticipated benefits and potential hazards of the study and the discomfort it may entail).

4.4 Free power of choice: The prospective subject or proxy is in no way highly dependent upon those who would be seeking consent.

4.5 Person or proxy maintains the right to withdraw at any time without prejudice.

4.6 Person or proxy will be informed that results of the study will be made available to him/her upon request.

4.7 In instances of nontherapeutic experimentation, the proxy can give his consent only if the experiment entails no significant risk to the person's well-being. Moreover, the greater the person's incompetency and vulnerability, the greater the reasons must be to perform any medical experimentation, especially nontherapeutic.

5) Equitable selection of subjects

5.1 Patient population: Distribution of subjects is randomized and not solely those who are less advantaged.

5.2 Protection of the vulnerable: no use of institutionalized subjects (prisoners) or persons with limited capacities to consent.

5.3 Subjects should be volunteers.

5.4 Subjects should be protected from arbitrary turn down without criteria.

6) Compensation for research-related injury

6.1 Provision exists to discontinue research that is determined to likely result in injury, disability or death to the experimental subject.

6.2 Subjects who suffer physical, psychological or social injury in the course of research shall be compensated 1) if the injury is primarily caused by such research and 2) if the injury exceeds that reasonably associated with such illness from which the subject may be suffering, as well as with treatment usually associated with such illness at the time the subject began participating in the research. (5)

From an ethical point of view, this IRB Worksheet is noteworthy in starting out with four fundamental ethical principles (beneficence, nonmaleficence, respecting persons, and justice) and deriving from them six more specific norms for evaluating proposed research projects (good research design, balance of harm and benefit, competence of the investigators, informed consent, equitable selection of subjects, and compensation for research-related injury). Exactly how do the six norms follow from the four fundamental principles?

The norms of good research design and competence of the investigator(s) are related to the principle of beneficence. For "without a competent investigator (or investigative team) and good research design, there will be no benefits forthcoming from the study." (6) These two norms are also related to the principle of nonmaleficence. This is so because "competent investigators and good research design also protect subjects from harm." (6) Further, "the requirements that the investigator(s) be competent and the research well designed serve to ensure that people's time is not wasted and that their desire to participate in a meaningful activity is not frustrated." (6) These two norms also uphold the principle of respect for persons. (6)

The norm of balancing harm and benefit is derived from both the principle of beneficence (doing good) and the principle of nonmaleficence (avoiding harm).

The principle of respecting persons comes from the philosopher Immanuel Kant and "requires that persons not be used merely as a means to another's end." (6) The norm of informed consent upholds this principle by ensuring that research subjects "are not 'used' by another without their knowledge and consent." (6)

The principle of justice requires fairness in the distribution of benefits and of burdens. Justice is the foundation for the norm requiring an equitable selection of subjects. The "burdens" of research activity are the risks involved in experimentation, and it would be unfair to make the less advantaged and the vulnerable in society take all the risks. Obviously, the principle of justice also serves as the foundation for the norm concerning compensation for research-related injury.

How does the blood pressure medication research project at Sun Valley Care Center stand up against these norms (and the more specific criteria for implementing them)? While we will not comment on each of the specific criteria listed in the IRB Worksheet, there are several points that stand out and deserve comment.

Balancing Benefits and Risks

Any research project involves a balancing of benefits and risks for the human subjects participating in it (see IRB Worksheet 2.2). This is clearly illustrated in the case of Sun Valley Care Center. The occupational therapist Marilyn Stewart is cautioned by Sun Valley's administrator to watch for unusual symptoms or behavior in residents that may be caused by the medication being tested. These possible undesirable effects constitute the risks of this particular research study. These risks are counterbalanced by the expected benefits of the new medication; namely, that the residents will experience fewer of the unpleasant side effects of the currently standard blood pressure medications.

Participation in this research project may also have benefits for the residents of Sun Valley Care Center that are less obvious:

> Very few people have discussed the benefits of being a research subject. We might consider that to open up nursing homes and other long-term care settings to competent and humane research could offer many benefits, such as increased social interaction, increased interest in the problems of the people who are in that environment, and a sense of meaning. One of the problems of chronic and incurable disease is that we really don't have an existential explanation that gives people a meaning to their suffering if we can't cure it. One of the ways to give meaning to an experience is to make a person feel that he or she is participating in a human endeavor in which they're not alone. Many of the people who are residents in long-term care facilities like to feel that they are making some contribution to the future, to society, and give meaning to their remaining lives in this way. By refusing to do research in those settings, we deny them that option. (7)

In sum, it is suggested that the very fact of being involved in a research project, independent of the medical information to be gained through that project, can bring benefits to residents of long-term care facilities. Research projects can call attention to and address problems encountered in the long-term care setting. Residents of long-term care facilities often suffer from loneliness because they do not have family and friends visiting them. Participation in a research project can increase the opportunities for social interaction available to such residents. Most especially, participation in research projects can give residents a sense of making a contribution to the lives of other people, which in turn gives meaning to their own lives and the suffering they may be experiencing.

Equitable Selection of Subjects

In the past there has been a problem with persons living in an institutional setting, such as a long-term care facility, being used as research subjects as a matter of convenience:

> Historically, nursing home patients were used as research participants disproportionately to their representation in the population, as were prisoners and other institutionalized groups, primarily for the convenience of the investigator. If the researcher can get all the subjects in one place, it is much easier to collect samples, do interviews, or conduct follow-up of the research. For example, it was much easier to get the consent of prisoners to participate by giving trivial amounts of money (or in some cases cartons of cigarettes) than it would have been to obtain consent from people in the community who have greater freedom. The studies were not particularly or especially relevant to problems of prisoners or problems of nursing home patients and therefore it was thought that this kind of selection bias was inequitable. (8)

Since medical research benefits society as a whole, there should, as a matter of justice, be an "equitable distribution of the burdens of participation in research." (8)

This entails that "populations not be selected simply for the convenience of the investigator, but that they be selected for true representativeness related to the sample selection needs of the study." (8) Thus one criterion of legitimate research and experimentation is that subjects be selected equitably. No one group of persons should be used exclusively since this involves the possibility of exploiting certain groups in society, especially those who are less advantaged (see IRB Worksheet 5.1).

As far as we know, the new blood pressure medication is being tested only at Sun Valley Care Center. If Sun Valley were a county facility for indigent elderly persons (versus a nursing home that includes residents who pay their own expenses), we would have good reason to worry that the research project was "using" poor people. However, we have no reason to think that Sun Valley is this type of facility. At the same time, we may worry that only the residents of Sun Valley are subjects in the research study. Are they being taken advantage of because they are in a nursing home? Why does the research study not include some elderly persons still living at home? (7)

Free and Informed Consent

Occupational therapist Marilyn Stewart notes a concern about the level of understanding the residents have of the project in which they are participating. This raises the issue of the residents' ability to give free and informed consent to participation in the research project.

A prominent principle in contemporary health care ethics is *autonomy*. Autonomy refers to self-determination. The principle of autonomy affirms the right of an individual to make the final decision in matters pertaining to his or her own life, including his or her health care. The requirement to obtain the free and informed consent of an individual to participate in research and experimentation (see IRB Worksheet 4.1-4.4) is often grounded in the principle of autonomy as well as in the principle of respect for persons.

According to standards for long-term care developed by the Joint Commission on Accreditation of Healthcare Organizations (JCAHO), "the resident has the right to participate or not to participate in research, investigation, or clinical trials"[RI.3.1]. (9) Participation in research should never be a condition for admission to a facility, nor should a facility require a blanket consent statement on admission for research participation [Intent of RI.3.1]. (9) Rather, consent by the resident (or the resident's proxy decision maker) should be required prior to each research project [Intent of RI.3.1]. (9) The procedure of obtaining informed consent should involve giving a clear and concise explanation of the resident's condition, of the proposed treatment or procedure, of the potential benefits, risks, and alternatives of the proposed treatment or procedure, and of any costs to be borne by the resident [RI.2.18]. (9) It is standard practice that a potential research subject (or his proxy) sign a consent form to participate in the research project.

In general, there are challenges to obtaining truly free and informed consent from individuals to participate in research projects. One challenge is using language that is understandable to the potential research subjects in the consent forms that they must sign. Many consent forms "require the potential volunteer to 'synthesize information from complex or lengthy passages'...or to 'make high-level inferences or use specialized background knowledge' about medicine...." (10) Based on the results of the National Adult Literacy Survey (1993), it is estimated that only 3 percent to 20 percent of American adults have the reading skills needed to understand current research consent forms. (10) Moreover, the survey indicated that people with a chronic illness, disability, or impairment have even lower levels of literacy skills than the total sample. (10) This finding is especially relevant to the case involving the residents of Sun Valley Care Center in evaluating their ability to give informed consent to participation in the blood pressure medication research project.

As an illustration of the problem about using understandable language, consider the following excerpt from a consent form for trial of a new drug (IND):

> You will initially receive 50 milligrams (mg) of [IND] per kilogram (kg) of your body weight, followed by 25 mg/kg every 6 hours for 4 days, followed by 12.5 mg/kg every 6 hours for 6 days. (10)

This statement is not likely to give any clear information about dosage levels to someone who is not a health care worker. Consider a possible revision of it:

> The first dose will start right away. We will give bigger doses in the first 4 days, and smaller doses the last 6 days. Those are the same doses used for many years to treat other diseases. (10)

Not only is the language here much simpler and less technical, but the revision has the advantage of addressing a question potential research subjects will probably have. Few subjects are likely to want to know exactly how many milligrams of an experimental drug they will receive. They are more likely to want to know whether the dosage level is itself part of the experiment or if the same dose was found effective in previous research. The revision answers this question in a clear and straightforward way. (10)

Other problems with obtaining truly free and informed consent concern the amount and nature of the information that is communicated. Studies indicate that the longer the consent form, the smaller the number of people that read the form in its entirety. This results in less, rather than more, information being conveyed. (10) Further, extensive detail "usually enhances the subject's confusion." (11) Again, studies indicate that the more elaborate the material presented to potential research subjects, the less they understand. (11) Indeed, an investigator "conceivably could exploit his authority and knowledge and extract 'informed consent' by overwhelming the candidate-subject with information." (11) Researchers face the challenge of constructing consent forms that contain all the essential information but still are concise and relatively brief.

It has also been found that the procedure of "next day consent" improves the communication process. Soliciting consent takes place in a two-stage process, spread over at least twenty-four hours. This gives time for more information to be absorbed by potential research subjects and for discussion with their family members. (10)

As well as these challenges to obtaining free and informed consent, there are problems specific to the long-term care context. For one thing, long-term care facilities (like Sun Valley Care Center in our case) are *total institutions* within which "all aspects of a person's life are connected with the social structure." (1) In turn, there can be social forces operating to encourage and pressure a resident or patient to do what is expected of him or her. (1) For example, the consent process for a resident "may be influenced by the subject's desire to please the caregiver and thus to continue a positive relationship." (8) Further, "the closeness and lack of privacy" found in most institutions "may easily lead to a kind of 'group think' or pressure from peers to participate or not." (7) In one recorded case, "peer pressure apparently kept persons from agreeing to join in a rather innocuous study" in a nursing home. (8)

Residents of long-term care facilities can suffer from physical impairments that interfere with the consent process. For example, some of the residents of Sun Valley Care Center have poor eyesight and are hard of hearing. In this case, the communication process for obtaining a research subject's consent can be enhanced through the use of such items as portable flip cards that summarize key points in large print and contain graphics and diagrams. (10)

Residents with mental impairments present a more difficult problem. If a resident is clearly incapacitated mentally, there is no question but that resort must be made to a proxy decision maker for consent to participation in a research project. Residents suffering from mild to moderate dementia present the difficult case:

> In this group, personality and expression of preference is largely maintained, no guardian is necessary, and many decisions the person makes are respected. Memory may be severely impaired, however, and their judgments may not seem reasonable to us. Should we then allow such persons to agree to participate in research? Can we measure competence by mental status examinations? Cognitive testing, especially with ill people, is not an adequate measure of the entire range of the human personality involved in a value decision. (7)

Similarly, questions have arisen about the ability of persons with deficits in short-term memory to consent to participation in research projects:

> Professionals have legal concerns if the patient doesn't remember consenting. On the other hand, if one knows that the person understands during the interaction and if he gives the consent freely, does the fact that he can't remember doing so the next day invalidate his decision? Many empirical studies of informed consent demonstrate that even normal people don't remember what they are told during the consent interview. Are we unduly penalizing the elderly by requiring them to remember what normal persons cannot? (7)

One physician has suggested the following guidelines for determining the ability of a resident of a long-term care facility to consent to participation in a research project:

- In determining capacity, the assessment of a resident's actual functioning in decision making situations should be weighed more heavily than a specific score on a mental status exam. Such assessment requires the involvement of someone who has some experience over time with the resident.

- Whenever possible, the resident's physician and a family member or close friend should be included in early discussions about the research project. These individuals can contribute to the assessment of the resident's level of understanding of the project and to the consistency of the resident's decision with his other values and decisions.

- A lesser standard of intellectual understanding may be acceptable to use in the case of residents of a long-term care facility. This is because of the apparent phenomenon of less complete understanding of scientific material by elderly subjects even without cognitive impairment.

- Studies involving minimal risk to residents (for example, observation in otherwise public situations, interviews without heavily emotional content, noninvasive medical studies using hair, fingernails, urine or blood samples taken for another purpose) may require less stringent criteria of cognitive function than studies involving greater risk or intrusiveness. (8)

Proxy Consent for Participation in Research and Experimentation

In our case, occupational therapist Marilyn Stewart notes that some of the residents of Sun Valley Care Center who are subjects in the blood pressure medication experiment are suffering from dementia, in varying degrees. Some of them may not have the capacity themselves to give free and informed consent to participation in the research project. Indeed, Marilyn raises the question of who made the decision about the residents participating in it.

In the case of mentally incapacitated adults and in the case of minors, proxy consent is recognized as legitimate. This is indicated in the IRB Worksheet presented above: "Person involved has legal capacity to give consent (OR if person is legally incompetent, guardian consent; OR if a minor, responsible relative consent in addition to minor consent)" (4.2). However, some ethicists draw a distinction between *consenting for oneself* and the role of *consenting for another*, placing restrictions on the latter type of consent.

Medical research and experimentation is considered therapeutic if it has the potential to benefit the subjects participating in the project. On the other hand, research and experimentation is classified as nontherapeutic if it is not expected to benefit the subjects themselves but will allow the researchers to gain knowledge that will be of benefit to other patients. Some ethicists hold that proxy decision makers cannot licitly give consent to research and experimentation that is nontherapeutic in character. (1, 12) Their reasoning is that a proxy decision maker has a duty to act in the best interests of the person he represents and for the welfare of that person. (1, 12) Other ethicists take a less restrictive position, allowing for proxy consent to research and experimentation that poses only minimal risk to the subject. (12) The IRB Worksheet given above allows for proxy consent for nontherapeutic research and experimentation, with certain qualifications: "In instances of nontherapeutic experimentation, the proxy can give his consent only if the experiment entails no significant risk to the person's well-being. Moreover, the greater the person's incompetency and vulnerability, the greater the reasons must be to perform any medical experimentation, especially nontherapeutic" (4.7).

These stipulations and restrictions do not pose any problem for the research project being carried on at Sun Valley Care Center. The new blood pressure medication being tested is expected to have fewer of the unpleasant side effects many older persons experience with the currently standard medications. If the new medication works as expected, it will clearly be of benefit to those taking it. Thus this project qualifies as therapeutic research for the residents participating in the project. Even those residents suffering from dementia may be included in the project, with the consent of the appropriate proxy decision maker.

FOR GROUP DISCUSSION

1. You are the administrator in a long-term care facility with a special Alzheimer's unit. A nursing student from a nearby college asks you if he can conduct a research project in that unit. The research project will consist simply in playing tapes of Gregorian chant for two hours a day in the unit for a month and observing the residents to determine if the music has a calming effect on their behavior. How do you respond to this request? Would you feel comfortable in granting permission yourself for this project? If not, what procedures would you follow?

2. Complaints have been voiced about the slowness of the U.S. Food and Drug Administration (FDA) in testing and approving new drugs. Should a terminally ill patient be allowed to have any drug he might wish to try, even if research and testing on it have not yet been completed? Should we be guided in these decisions by the ethical principle of autonomy or the ethical principle of nonmaleficence? (13)

3. It is possible to sustain by technological means the vital functions of an individual who has suffered brain death. It has been proposed that such legally dead human beings be sustained specifically for use as subjects in medical research experiments. (14, 15, 16) From an ethical point of view, do you see any problems with doing this?

NOTES

1. "Medical Experimentation and Informed Consent" in Ronald Munson (ed.), *Intervention and Reflection Basic Issues in Medical Ethics*, 5th ed. (Belmont, CA: Wadsworth, 1996).
2. A.M. Capron, "Human Experimentation" in Robert M. Veatch (ed.), *Medical Ethics* (Boston: Jones & Bartlett, 1989).
3. *Trials of War Criminals before the Nuremberg Military Tribunals under Control Council Law No. 10*, vol. 2 (Washington, D.C.: United States Government Printing Office, 1949).

4. Adopted by the 18th World Medical Assembly, Helsinki, Finland, 1964; revised 1975, 1983, 1989. Reprinted in the *Encyclopedia of Bioethics* rev. ed. (New York: Macmillan, 1995).

5. *Research Manual*, Mercy Health Center, Dubuque, IA (1996).

6. Robert J. Levine & Karen Lebacqz, "Ethical Considerations in Clinical Trials," *Clinical Pharmacology and Therapeutics* 25/5-2 (May 1979).

7. Christine K. Cassel, "Research in Nursing Homes Ethical Issues," *Journal of the American Geriatrics Society* 33/11 (Nov.1985): 795-99.

8. Christine Cassel, "Ethical Issues in the Conduct of Research in Long Term Care," *The Gerontologist* 28 Suppl. (1988): 90-6.

9. Joint Commission on Accreditation of Healthcare Organizations, 2002-2003 *Standards for Long Term Care* (Oakbrook Terrace, IL: Joint Commission Resources, 2002).

10. William L. Freeman, "Making Research Consent Forms Informative and Understandable: The Experience of the Indian Health Service," *Cambridge Quarterly of Healthcare Ethics* 3 (1994): 510-21.

11. F.J. Ingelfinger, "Informed (But Uneducated) Consent," *New England Journal of Medicine* 287/9 (Aug. 31, 1972): 465-66.

12. Benedict M. Ashley, O.P. & Kevin D. O'Rourke, O.P., *Healthcare Ethics A Theological Analysis*, 3rd ed. (St. Louis: Catholic Health Association, 1989).

13. "Drug Testing, Autonomy, and Access to Unapproved Drugs" in Ronald Munson (ed.), *Intervention and Reflection Basic Issues in Medical Ethics*, 5th ed. Belmont, CA: Wadsworth, 1996).

14. Willard Gaylin, "Harvesting the Dead," *Harpers* 249 (Sept. 1974): 23-6.

15. R. Carson, J. Frias & R. Melker, "Case Study: Research with Brain-Dead Children," *IRB* 3/1 (1981): 5-6.

16. S. Martyn, "Using the Brain Dead for Medical Research," *Utah Law Review* (1986): 1-28.

FOR FURTHER STUDY

• A.M. Capron, "Human Experimentation" in Robert M. Veatch (ed.), *Medical Ethics*, 2nd ed. (Sudbury, MA: Jones & Bartlett, 1997).

• Gregory E. Pence, *Classic Cases in Medical Ethics Accounts of Cases That Have Shaped Medical Ethics, with Philosophical, Legal, and Historical Backgrounds*, 2nd ed. (New York: McGraw-Hill, 1995), Chapter 9, "Human Subjects: The Tuskegee Syphilis Study."

• Thomas A. Mappes and David DeGrazia (eds.), *Biomedical Ethics*, 4th ed. (New York: McGraw-Hill, 1996), Chapter 4, "Human and Animal Experimentation." This chapter contains codes of research ethics and papers on historical and cultural causes for concern about human experimentation, proxy consent for children and the incompetent elderly, and experimental design and randomized clinical trials.

• John W. Warren et al., "Informed Consent by Proxy An Issue in Research with Elderly Patients," *New England Journal of Medicine* 315/18 (Oct. 30, 1986): 1124-8.

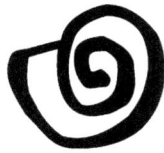

Chapter 20

Allocating Resources in Health Care

Many more individuals can be in need of health care than we have resources available. One obvious example is organ transplantation. Thousands of individuals are on waiting lists to get an organ transplant, and many will die before an organ becomes available to them.

Hard choices must be made concerning how we distribute our health care resources. These decisions arise on several levels.

The term *macroallocation* refers to decisions concerning types of services provided. For example, should the local community hospital expand its services for cardiac care or establish a cancer center? Should a long-term care facility expand its skilled nursing unit or establish an adult day care center? Questions of macroallocation can also arise at the societal and governmental levels. How much funding should go to research on AIDS versus research on Alzheimer's disease? If we were to establish a national health care plan, which services should everyone be guaranteed to receive under the plan, and which services might be available only to those who can afford them personally?

The term *microallocation* refers to decisions about distributing resources among individual patients and residents. The resources in question include both medical treatments and the services and time of health care workers. Suppose, for example, that Michael, 76, and Greg, 45, are both in need of a heart transplant and one heart becomes available. Which one should receive this scarce resource? Or suppose that a nursing home resident, Joyce, has terminal pancreatic cancer and that her family wants "everything done," including transferring her to the hospital and placing her in the intensive care unit (ICU). If physicians believe that ICU care would prolong Joyce's life for a few days at most, should the resources of the ICU be spent on Joyce's care? Or, on a more mundane level, suppose that three residents in the skilled nursing unit of a long-term care facility all put on the call light at the same time but that there is only one staff person available to answer the calls. Who should be the first one to receive a response?

Ethically, these questions involve *distributive justice;* that is, fairness in the distribution of benefits and resources. In this chapter, we will discuss one case at the level of microallocation and two cases at the level of macroallocation pertaining to long-term care.

Specifically, this chapter covers:
- *principles that health care workers may use in deciding how to allocate their time and services among various residents;*
- *principles for making decisions about the types of services a health care facility should provide;*
- *age-based rationing of health care.*

CASE STUDY

Barbara Stock is a physical therapist who comes weekly to Wesley Manor to provide physical therapy services for its residents. Wesley Manor is a multi-level facility for retired persons consisting of independent living apartments, assisted living units, and a nursing home unit.

Barbara is currently providing physical therapy for three residents, Wanda Taylor, Fred Sullivan, and George Kohl. Before she visits these residents, she stops by the office of the Director of Nursing (DON) to get an update on their conditions.

Wanda is residing in the independent living apartments. The DON tells Barbara that Wanda's daughter is making a trip today from another state to see her mother and bringing her children with her. They plan to take Wanda out to lunch. Because of the long driving distance, they're not sure exactly what time they will arrive that morning.

Fred is in the nursing home unit. The DON tells Barbara that Fred has been experiencing considerable discomfort in his left leg for several days to the point of needing additional pain medication. The DON hopes that physical therapy will make him more comfortable.

George resides in the assisted living unit. George is the kind of person who has gone by a schedule all his life. He gets very upset when things get "off schedule," and this emotional stress aggravates his problem with high blood pressure. George is normally the first resident that Barbara treats, promptly at 11:00 A.M.

While Barbara is having this conversation with the Director of Nursing, the DON receives a call that a resident, Amanda Miller, has choked on a piece of hard candy she wasn't supposed to have in the first place, and that she has stopped breathing. Resuscitation is needed immediately. Barbara has been trained in CPR.

To which resident should Barbara give attention first? In what order should the rest be treated?

Allocating Staff Time and Services Among Residents

The time and services of health care workers are resources that must sometimes be allocated. Especially when there is a staffing shortage, health care workers may be faced with decisions about which patient or resident should receive care first. Ethically, these allocation decisions involve *distributive justice*, the principle concerned with fairness in the distribution of benefits and resources.

Philosophers have tried to spell out more concretely how benefits and resources are distributed fairly. One interpretation given to distributive justice is the *principle of equality*, according to which "everyone is to be treated the same in all respects." (1) More simply stated, this interpretation of distributive justice maintains that "everyone is entitled to the same size slice of the pie." (1) Another interpretation of distributive justice is the *principle of contribution*, according to which "everyone should get back that proportion of social goods that is the result of his or her productive labor." (1) If one person works twice as hard or long as a second, the first person should be entitled to twice as large a share in the benefits. (1) The interpretation of distributive justice that is most likely relevant to the situation of health care workers is the *principle of need*:

> The principle of need is an extension of the egalitarian principle of equal distribution. If goods are parceled out according to individual need, those who have greater needs will receive a greater share. However, the outcome will be one of equality. Since the basic needs of everyone will be met, everyone will end up at the same level. The treatment of individuals will be equal, in this respect, even though the proportion of goods they receive will not be. (1)

Thus, if two (or more) residents need attention, a health care worker should prioritize her services and time according to which patient has the greater (greatest) need.

Let us apply the principle of need to the decisions Barbara Stock has to make. First, Barbara has to decide between giving physical therapy to Wanda, Fred, and George (the reason she came to Wesley Manor) and administering CPR to Amanda, the resident who choked on a piece of candy. Amanda is in a life-threatening situation while Wanda, Fred, and George are not. Clearly, the resident who choked and needs resuscitation has the greatest need. If no one else who is adequately trained in CPR is immediately available, Barbara should respond to Amanda first.

The problem is that many decisions about allocating time and services are not this clear cut. Consider the decision Barbara has to make after she has administered CPR to Amanda. George is probably already upset that Barbara is late to administer his physical therapy, and this is not good for his blood pressure. While George is experiencing emotional distress, Fred has been experiencing serious physical discomfort. Physical therapy may well help relieve the discomfort he has been experiencing for several days. On the other hand, if Barbara does not attend to Wanda right away, her daughter may come to take her to lunch before Barbara can get to her. If Wanda misses her physical therapy entirely, this is likely to result in physical discomfort for her later in the week. Which of these residents should Barbara attend to first? Whose need is the greatest?

If Fred is presently experiencing serious discomfort, we would likely judge his need to be the greatest. On the other hand, if his discomfort is being adequately managed through pain medication, he could probably wait a bit to have his physical therapy administered.

We might then consider the needs of Wanda to be the most urgent. After all, it may be a case of Wanda receiving therapy now or forgoing it entirely for that week. George will eventually receive his therapy; the only question is when.

At the same, George's emotional distress cannot be totally discounted. Indeed, this may aggravate his high blood pressure. George too has a real need.

In this case, a solution might be found that meets the needs of both Wanda and George. Before seeing Wanda, perhaps Barbara could stop into George's room to calm him down by explaining to him the incident about the resident choking and needing CPR, and reassuring him that she will be back to administer his therapy as soon as she is able.

CASE STUDY

St. Mary's Care Center has just received a gift of $150,000 from the estate of a life-long donor. The development office is preparing a recommendation to the Center's board of trustees on how the money should be used.

One proposal under consideration, put forward by St. Mary's dietary staff, is to use the money to remodel the resident dining area from cafeteria-style service to a more elegant restaurant style dining room. This would create a much more pleasant atmosphere for the facility's 125 residents. The dietary staff points out that other area long-term care facilities have already adopted this style for their food service, and that such a dining room would make residency at St. Mary's much more attractive to potential residents and family members who come to tour the facility.

Another proposal is to use the money to finish part of the basement area of the facility to be used for an adult day care center. This proposal has been put forward by St. Mary's activity director as well as by one of the facility's social workers. They point out that there are no adult day care services currently available in the community, and that such a center is likely to attract at least 35 clients a day. Further, an adult day care center will allow its clients to remain at home for a longer period of time rather than having to enter a nursing home, which will represent cost savings for all concerned. The clients of the adult day care center will be provided with health care services and opportunities for socialization not available in their homes. And the families of the clients will also benefit through respite from their caregiving responsibilities.

Which project, the dining area or the adult day care center, should be funded?

Deciding on Types of Services Offered by a Health Care Facility

In this case the ethical theory of *utilitarianism* might be called on to guide decision making. Utilitarianism is often characterized as the principle of "the greatest good for the greatest number." More exactly, a utilitarian makes judgments on the basis of consequences of action, taking into account all who will be affected by what is done. The right action to perform is the one that will have the best consequences overall, when the effects (both positive and negative) for everyone concerned are considered and evaluated.

In making the decision whether to fund remodeling of the dining area or of the basement to create space for an adult day care center, a utilitarian would try to determine which option will have the best consequences overall for residents, the facility's staff, the facility itself, and members of the community that the facility serves. How many people will be served by a renovated dining area, and how many will be served by an adult day care center? What degree of benefit will residents, elderly persons, and their families receive from each of the projects? How will the quality of life for residents be enhanced by a renovated dining area, and how does this compare with the enhanced quality of life made possible for the patrons of the adult day care center and their family caregivers? What impact will each of the projects have on the working conditions of the facility's staff? Will either project create new job opportunities? Which project will be more profitable for the facility, thus helping to ensure its continued financial viability? These are the kinds of questions that a utilitarian would ask in making a decision between the two projects.

Not all ethicists, however, are utilitarians. They maintain that there are values other than the positive and negative consequences of an action that should be taken into account in determining rightness and wrongness of action.

For example, some believe that health care is basically a human and community service. As such, meeting the health care needs of the people in its service area must be one of the guiding principles of a facility's operation. In the case about St. Mary's Care Center, there are currently no adult day care services available within the community. According to this viewpoint, the fact that adult day care services are an unmet need within the community constitutes in itself a reason for St. Mary's Care Center to invest in initiating such a project.

Some health care facilities, especially those with a religious sponsorship, may go even further and see an obligation to meet the health care needs of the poor and of those without adequate health insurance. (2) For these facilities, this special commitment will also direct decisions about the types of services in which they invest their resources. Thus, for example, the number of low income persons who would be served by an adult day care center versus the number served as residents of St. Mary's would be a factor in which project to fund.

CASE STUDY

It is the year 2010. Rita Meier, a retired high school history teacher, has been a resident of Maple Grove Care Center for a year and a half. She has just turned eighty. The bones in both her knees have badly degenerated, making it very difficult for her to walk, even with the assistance of a walker. This is what caused her to give up her home and become a resident of Maple Grove.

Rita is still very alert mentally. She is an avid reader and likes listening to music. She makes a point of keeping up on current events through news programs on the television and radio, and discusses them with other residents and with staff. She immensely enjoys her four great-grandchildren when they come to visit her. She is the leader of the bible study group at Maple Grove. In spite of her physical limitations in walking, Rita still enjoys life.

During her routine annual physical exam, it is discovered that Rita has breast cancer. The cancer, however, is still in its early stages. It could be treated through surgery followed by chemotherapy. Rita tells her physician that she is ready and willing to begin treatment—the sooner the better—so that she can get on with her life.

Rita, however, is on Medicaid. Her physician, Dr. Boyle, informs her that Medicaid will not pay for cancer treatments for anyone over the age of 78. Dr. Boyle tells her that he is sorry, but that governmental policy simply will not allow him to provide cancer treatments for someone her age. He assures her that pain medication will be provided to keep her comfortable.

Rita begins crying. "I'm not ready to die," she tells Dr. Boyle. "I still have too much living to do."

Age-Based Rationing of Health Care

Philosopher Daniel Callahan has created a controversy by advocating age-based rationing of health care. According to Callahan's proposal, medical treatments and technologies that extend life would not be available to individuals past a certain age as a matter of social policy. Such procedures and treatments as organ transplants, kidney dialysis, chemotherapy, resuscitation, mechanical ventilation, antibiotics, and artificial nutrition and hydration might well be automatically denied to individuals past the given age limit. In the hypothetical case of Rita Meier, such a social policy would deny her treatment for breast cancer for no other reason than her age.

In developing his proposal Callahan uses the concept of a natural life span which represents living a full life:

> We need a notion of a full life that is based on some deeper understanding of human need and sensible possibility, not the latest state of medical technology or medical possibility. We should instead think of natural life span as the achievement of a life long enough to accomplish, for the most part, those opportunities that life typically affords people and which we ordinarily take to be the prime benefits of enjoying a life at all—that of loving and living, of raising a family, of finding and carrying out work that is satisfying, of reading and thinking, and of cherishing our friends and families.
>
> If we envisioned a natural life span that way, then we could begin to intensify the devising of ways to get people to that stage of life, and to work to make certain they do so in good health and social dignity. People will differ on what they may count as a natural life span; determining its appropriate range for social policy purposes would need extended thought and debate. My own view is that it can now be achieved by the late 70s or early 80s. (3)

Callahan then suggests three principles for limiting access to health care for older persons, at least under governmentally sponsored programs:

- Government has a duty, based on our collective social obligations to each other, to help people live out a natural life span, but not actively to help medically extend life beyond that point.

- Government is obliged to develop and pay for only that kind and degree of life-extending technology necessary for medicine to achieve and serve the end of a natural life span.

- Beyond the point of natural life span, government should provide only the means necessary for the relief of suffering, not life-extending technology. (3)

In Callahan's view, "the future goal of medicine in the care of the aged should be that of improving the quality of their lives, not in seeking ways to extend their lives." (3)

Economic considerations are part of the motivation for proposing age-based rationing of health care. The number of older persons in the population is increasing, and they need a substantial amount of expensive health care services. Limiting the health care services available to this population is a way of relieving economic burdens on families and on society. (3, 4)

Economics is not the only factor involved in proposals for age-based rationing. Callahan believes that we need to regain a sense of our human mortality. The attempt to extend life indefinitely, according to Callahan, "fails to accept aging and death as part of the human condition." (3) Further, he thinks that the attempt to extend life indefinitely "fails to present to younger generations a model of wise stewardship." (3) In addition, it has been suggested that "the cultural value placed on youth in the United States also makes an increasing emphasis on an age criterion likely." (5) Indeed, Callahan himself says of the elderly that "their primary orientation should be to the young and the generations to come, not to their own age group." (3)

Callahan's proposal has met with vigorous criticism. For one thing, his proposal for age-based rationing is intended to apply to "life-extending technology," but one physician has noted the difficulties in clearly marking off this category of treatments:

> How are we to distinguish between life-extending care and life-improving technologies? For example, a ninety-nine-year-old patient who develops syncope (fainting spells) is admitted to the hospital and found to have periodic interruption of the heart rhythms during which time she passes out. She lives alone, has very severe arthritis, but no other serious illnesses. The treatment of choice for her heart disease (conduction system disorder) is a pacemaker. Without the pacemaker, we will send her home to continue fainting and falling. Either she will fall, break a hip, and lie there until she dies of dehydration, or she will be admitted to the orthopedic service, where at great cost and very poor likely outcome, the broken hip will be tended. The alternative is to give her a pacemaker, which will not only improve the quality of her life by preventing these things from happening but will also extend her life. How are we to make such a decision according to Callahan's proposed scheme? (6)

Addressing the economic argument for age-based rationing of health care, another line of criticism contends that the amount of money spent on health care is not disproportionate in comparison with other ways in which Americans spend their money:

> Two billion dollars per year is spent on renal dialysis; a similar amount on coronary artery bypass grafts. One is clearly a lifesaving treatment; the other is lifesaving only in a minority of cases. Is this too much to spend in either case, in a country that spends $3 billion annually on potato chips? (6)

Further, Callahan's proposal would change the very nature of medical practice. It would require physicians "to transfer their primary responsibility from the patient to the community, as represented by some kind of government regulatory function." (6) It would give over "to the state the basic function of medical decision-making for an entire group of patients." (6)

The above case study on age-based rationing involves denial of life-prolonging treatment for cancer to a woman. It has been pointed out that aged-based rationing of health care would affect elderly women more drastically than elderly men:

> While the ratio of elderly men to elderly women in 1960 was five to four, older women now outnumber older men three to two. More specifically, of those age sixty-five to seventy-four, 55 percent are women; of those seventy-five to eighty-four, 62 percent are women; of those over eighty-five, 71 percent are women. So if very elderly people are to be barred from lifesaving health care, it is predominantly women who are in view.

> If only publicly funded elderly patients are to go without lifesaving care, women are even more disproportionately affected. Elderly women are more likely than elderly men to live in poverty. In fact, 30 percent of women over eighty-five have incomes below the poverty line. Because they live longer than men (current life expectancies are about seventy-nine and seventy-two, respectively), they are more likely to exhaust their resources and less likely to have a spouse to care for them. A specific age cut-off for receiving lifesaving health care, then, will likely be set high enough to ensure a "full life" as life is typically experienced by men—implicitly devaluing the years beyond that point, which are primarily years of women's lives. (4)

One argument offered in favor of age-based rationing focuses on length of medical benefit. The premise is that "scarce resources should be given to those who will receive the greatest (i.e., longest) benefit if treated." (5) Since "the elderly will not live as long as younger patients and so will not receive as great a benefit," it is legitimate to allocate scarce medical resources on the basis of age. On the other hand, it is subjectively difficult to claim "that a longer life is more important to preserve than a shorter one" for the reason that "each person's life is uniquely important to that person." (5) Further, each person has an equal right to life, which entails "an equal right of all to have access to life (within limits), irrespective of each one's circumstances." (5) This right "does not diminish with age." (5)

Finally, we are asked to consider that age-based rationing of health care established for the sake of efficiency may have harmful effects on societal attitudes and values:

> There are other serious losses at issue here, however. One example is the dehumanizing effect of the justification's preoccupation with efficiency. In a way reminiscent of social-value considerations, it tends to favor efficiency over equal regard to persons. There is more to the health of a society, however, than physical well-being. The fairness and humaneness with which people are treated, among other things, are also critical. A society that ignores this in its pursuit of efficient medical care may stave off for a while the effects of illness, only to end up as a society incapacitated by inhumanity and insensitivity. (5)

The Council on Ethical and Judicial Affairs of the American Medical Association has taken the position that "decisions regarding the allocation of limited medical resources among patients should consider only ethically appropriate criteria relating to medical need" and that "non-medical criteria, such as...age...should not be considered." (7)

FOR GROUP DISCUSSION

1. Pamela Howard is the Director of Nursing at Bethany Home. Because of a flu epidemic in the community, only half of the nursing staff has been able to come to work today. Somehow she and the staff on duty managed to get all the residents dressed and down to breakfast, but she is now assessing how to allocate the available staff for the rest of the day. Pamela decides to make a list of the care needs that must be met: medications must be dispensed to the residents; call lights must be answered for toileting; fifteen residents are scheduled to receive baths today; one resident must be readied to travel to a clinic for a doctor's appointment. In addition, today is the day for the residents' monthly birthday party, but the activity director is also out sick. And a local pastor is coming for a weekly church service. These activities mean so much to the residents, but many of them need assistance in getting to them.

   If you were Pamela, how would you instruct the nursing staff to use and prioritize their time? And what are the reasons behind your advice?

2. Consider the case of St. Mary's Care Center, where a decision had to be made about how to use a $150,000 bequest from the estate of a life-long donor. The projects under consideration are, first, remodeling the residents' dining room, and second, remodeling a space to start an adult day care center. Suppose that you are a member of that facility's ethics committee and that the development office has asked the committee to make a recommendation about which project should be funded. Which project would you personally recommend, and why?

3. Suppose you are a legislator who has to vote on a proposal to give 5 million dollars to research projects to find a cure for AIDS. An alternate proposal would give the same amount of money to research on Alzheimer's disease. Which proposal would you vote for, and why? Is your decision influenced in any way by the fact that Alzheimer's disease affects older persons while AIDS is predominant among younger persons?

4. Richard Taylor, 80, is a resident of Brookhaven Village. He has serious heart problems, and ideally, he needs a heart transplant. Should he be put on the waiting list for a heart transplant when there are many other persons in need of a heart transplant, many of whom are considerably younger than Richard?

NOTES

1. "Principles of Distributive Justice" in Ronald Munson (ed.), *Intervention and Reflection Basic Issues in Medical Ethics*, 5th ed. (Belmont, CA: Wadsworth, 1996).
2. See, for example, the United States Conference of Catholic Bishops, *Ethical and Religious Directives for Catholic Health Care Services* (Washington, DC: United States Conference of Catholic Bishops, 2001). Available at http://www.nccbuscc.org
3. Daniel Callahan, "Aging and the Ends of Medicine," *Annals of the New York Academy of Sciences* 530 (June 15, 1988): 125-32. See also Daniel Callahan, *Setting Limits Medical Goals in an Aging Society* (New York: Simon & Schuster, 1987).
4. John F. Kilner, "Why Now? The Growing Interest in Limiting the Lifesaving Health Care Resources Available to Elderly People" in James W. Walters (ed.), *Choosing Who's to Live* (Urbana, IL: University of Illinois Press, 1996).
5. John F. Kilner, "Age Criteria in Medicine Are the Medical Justifications Ethical?" *Archives of Internal Medicine* 149 (Oct. 1989): 2343-6.
6. Christine K. Cassel, "The Limits of Setting Limits" in Paul Homer and Martha Holstein (eds.), *A Good Old Age?* (New York: Simon and Schuster, 1990).
7. Council on Ethical and Judicial Affairs of the American Medical Association, *Current Opinions* E-2.03 "Allocation of Limited Medical Resources." Available at http://www.ama-assn.org

FOR FURTHER STUDY

•   "Caring on Demand" in Rosalie A. Kane and Arthur L. Caplan (eds.), *Everyday Ethics Resolving Dilemmas in Nursing Home Life* (New York: Springer: 1990). This is a case study with commentary that raises issues about allocation of staff time and services.

•   Catholic Health Association of the United States, *With Justice for All? The Ethics of Healthcare Rationing* (St. Louis: Catholic Health Association of the United States, 1991). This pamphlet illustrates the values brought to decisions about the allocation of health care resources by one religious tradition.

•   Robert L. Barry and Gerard Bradley (eds.), *Set No Limits: A Rebuttal to Daniel Callahan's Proposal to Limit Health Care for the Elderly* (Urbana: University of Illinois Press, 1991).

- Kevin O'Rourke, "Ethical Issues in Resource Allocation in Health Care for the Elderly" in James C. Romeis, Rodney M. Coe, and John E. Morley (eds.), *Applying Health Services Research to Long Term Care* (New York: Springer, 1996).

- James J. Walters (ed.), *Choosing Who's to Live Ethics and Aging* (Urbana, IL: University of Illinois Press, 1996).

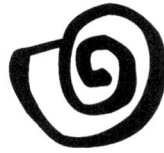

Chapter 21

Looking to the Future: Stem Cell Research

Some issues in health care ethics, such as confidentiality or forgoing life-sustaining treatments or resident rights, are perennial ones. Other issues emerge with the advent of new diseases (such as AIDS) or with new developments in scientific and medical research (such as the Human Genome Project). One issue that has recently become prominent, and that interfaces with public policy, is stem cell research.

This chapter covers:
* *biological facts about stem cells;*
* *potential uses for stem cells;*
* *the ethics of using aborted fetuses as a source of stem cells;*
* *ethical questions about using stem cells from early embryos;*
* *the controversy surrounding federal funding for embryonic stem cell research.*

CASE STUDY

It is the year 2015. Mr. Timothy Stern, aged 80, has been a resident at the Westridge Care Center for five years. After the death of his wife, he took up residency there because of limited mobility resulting from arthritis and, as he put it, from a "worn out" hip and knee. Within the last year, several members of the nursing staff have seen signs of dementia in him. His physician confirms that it is likely the beginning stage of Alzheimer's disease.

Sally Taylor, the administrator of Westridge, contacts Mr. Stern's daughter, Martha, about his condition. During a specially arranged care conference, Sally tells Martha that a new therapy is available that may reverse the dementia her father is beginning to experience. The therapy consists in implanting new brain tissue, grown from stem cells, into her father's brain. Sally assures Martha that this therapy has been well tested.

Initially, Martha is quite excited about the availability of a new therapy that could stop the progress of Alzheimer's disease in her father. Martha has a close friend whose mother suffered from Alzheimer's disease for ten years before her death, and she knows how devastating a disease it is.

At the same time, Martha remembers from her college biology course the controversy that surrounded the development of therapies from stem cells. Martha has always considered herself to be "pro-life," and she wonders about the ethics of using therapies dependent on stem cells. For this reason, she tells Sally Taylor that she wants to learn more about these therapies and to consult with her pastor before agreeing to the proposed treatment for her father.

What Are Stem Cells?

The various tissues and organs of the human body consist of specialized cells adapted to perform certain functions. *Stem cells* are cells that have the ability to reproduce themselves for long periods of time and to give rise to specialized cell types. While such cells as heart cells and skin cells are committed to conduct a specific function, a stem cell is uncommitted and remains this way until it receives a signal to develop into a specialized cell. (1)

Some stem cells are found in adults. An adult stem cell "is an undifferentiated (unspecialized) cell that occurs in a differentiated (specialized) tissue, renews itself, and becomes specialized to yield all of the specialized cell types of the tissue from which it originated." (1) Adult stems cells "are capable of making identical copies of themselves for the lifetime of the organism." (1) Sources of adult stem cells include "bone marrow, blood, the cornea and the retina of the eye, brain, skeletal muscle, dental pulp, liver, skin, the lining of the gastrointestinal tract, and pancreas." (1) Stem cells obtainable from umbilical cord blood and the placenta have also been placed in the category of "adult" stem cells. (2)

Stem cells have also been obtained from fetal tissue coming from aborted pregnancies. Technically called "embryonic germ cells," these stem cells are derived from the region of the fetus destined to develop into the testes or the ovaries. (1, 3)

Stem cells have been isolated from early stage human embryos. (1, 3) The process of obtaining embryonic stem cells typically begins with embryos produced through in vitro fertilization (IVF). Often "spare" frozen embryos are used; that is, embryos that a couple undergoing IVF have donated for research purposes because they have achieved the number of children they wish through IVF or because they have given up trying to have a child by this means. However, "research embryos" may be deliberately created to be a source of stem cells. (2, 4) At the blastocyst stage of its development, which occurs around day five, the early embryo contains two distinguishable structures: an "inner cell mass" which will develop into the fetus, and the "trophoblast" which will become the placenta. The trophoblast is removed from the embryo, the inner cell mass is isolated, and embryonic stem cells are extracted from the inner cell mass. The stem cells derived from the inner cell mass are then placed in culture. The intent is to coax these cells into differentiating into the desired tissue, which would then be placed into the tissue or organ of the recipient. (5)

However, such tissue or organ transplantation faces the well-known problem of immune rejection because the stem cells derived from embryos (or, for that matter, fetuses) would be genetically different from the recipient. One method for overcoming this problem, which researchers are exploring, is cloning. In a procedure known as "somatic cell nuclear transfer," an ovum that has had its nuclear DNA removed is combined with a somatic cell (a non-reproductive body cell) from a patient so that patient's set of genes is reprogrammed back to an embryonic state. When the appropriate stage of embryonic development is reached, the aforementioned procedure for obtaining stem cells would be used. This procedure is known as "therapeutic cloning" to distinguish it from the potential use of cloning to produce a child for a couple with infertility problems. (3, 6)

Use of Stem Cells in Research

Researchers are looking to stem cells as a way to replace cells and tissues in the body that are damaged or diseased in order to restore bodily functions. (1) Stem cells could potentially be used to grow nerve cells to repair spinal injuries and restore function to paralyzed limbs, and to grow heart muscle cells to replace useless scar tissue after a heart attack. Stem cells could potentially be used to make brain cells that would secrete dopamine for the treatment and control of Parkinson's disease, and to grow cells that make insulin to create a lifelong treatment for diabetes. They might be used to grow bone marrow to replace blood-forming organs damaged by disease or radiation, and in making blood cells that are genetically altered to resist a specific disease (such as HIV) to replace diseased blood cells. (7) Alzheimer's disease, end-stage kidney disease, liver failure, cancer, and multiple sclerosis are among the medical conditions for which stem cells might provide a therapy. (1)

There are yet other potential uses for stem cells. Embryonic stem cells are seen as potential research tools in "understanding fundamental events in embryonic development that one day may explain the causes of birth defects and approaches to correct or prevent them."(1) In the area of genetic medicine, stem cells are being "explored as a vehicle for delivering genes to specific tissues in the body." (1) In the area of pharmaceutical research, stem cells might be employed to develop specialized liver cells for the testing of new drugs. (1)

One important question being investigated and debated is whether stem cells from embryos, fetuses, and adults are equally useful for research and therapeutic purposes. For example, a report from the National Institutes of Health (July, 2001) has noted one difference:

> Human embryonic stem cells can be generated in abundant quantities in the laboratory and can be grown (allowed to proliferate) in their undifferentiated (or unspecialized) state for many, many generations. From a practical perspective in basic research or eventual clinical application, it is significant that millions of cells can be generated from one embryonic stem cell in the laboratory. In many cases, however, researchers have had difficulty finding laboratory conditions under which some adult stem cells can proliferate without becoming specialized. (1)

Embryonic stem cells and embryonic germ cells from fetuses also have the property of being pluripotent; that is, they have the ability to give rise to any type of specialized body cell. Adult stem cells are not pluripotent. However, adult stem cells may exhibit plasticity; that is, an adult stem cell from one tissue may have the ability to generate the specialized cell type of another tissue. For example, adult stem cells from bone marrow can generate cells that resemble neurons and other cell types commonly found in the brain. (1)

Some researchers point to various limitations of adult stem cells: stem cells from adults have not been isolated for all tissues of the body; they are often present in only minute quantities and are difficult to isolate and purify; their numbers decrease with age; they may contain genetic disorders and abnormalities. (3) Other researchers, however, point to success stories with the use of adult stem cells that have already taken place. (2, 8)

Thus, the aforementioned report from the National Institutes of Health gives the following assessment of the current state of research:

> For researchers and patients, there are many practical questions about stem cells that cannot yet be answered. How long will it take to develop therapies for Parkinson's disease and diabetes with and without human pluripotent stem cells? Can the full range of new therapeutic approaches be developed using only adult stem cells? ...Predicting the future of stem cell applications is impossible, particularly given the very early stage of the science of stem cell biology. To date, it is impossible to predict which stem cells—those derived from the embryo, the fetus, or the adult—or which methods of manipulating the cells, will best meet the needs of basic research and clinical applications. (1)

Accompanying this work on stem cell research is a vigorous ethical debate. The use of adult stem cells is generally uncontroversial, although it is sometimes forgotten that even here the ethical norms for legitimate research and experimentation on human beings must be observed (see chapter 19). The ethical controversy surrounds the use of stem cells derived from embryos (which are destroyed in the process of obtaining the stem cells) and from fetuses that have been electively aborted.

Ethics of Using Tissue from Aborted Fetuses

If someone believes that there are cases in which abortion is morally permissible, then using aborted fetuses as a source for stem cells is probably not troubling. Among those who believe that abortion is immoral, two schools of thought have emerged. The Human Fetal Tissue Transplantation Research Panel of the National Institutes of Health (NIH) has summarized these two positions in the following way:

> Abortion is immoral and so is the use of fetal tissue obtained thereby. No amount of good achieved in research or therapy could erase institutional complicity in the immorality of abortion itself or in encouragement of future abortions. No efforts at separating the procurement and use of fetal tissue from the abortion decision and procedure could make the use of fetal tissue from induced abortion morally acceptable.

> Abortion is immoral or undesirable, but as abortion is a legal procedure in our society and with appropriate safeguards can be separated from the subsequent research use of tissue derived therefrom, the use of fetal tissue in research and therapy is not seen as complicitous with the immorality of abortion. (9)

Among the safeguards suggested to separate the research use of fetal tissue from abortion are these stipulations:

- informed consent for research use of fetal tissue should be distinct from consent for the abortion and should be subsequent to it;

- even preliminary information about tissue donation should be withheld from the pregnant woman before she consents to the abortion;

- the procedure of abortion should be kept independent from the retrieval and use of fetal tissue;

- no financial compensation should be offered to the parents or to providers for aborted remains;

- parents should not be permitted to designate or to know the identity of the beneficiaries of their aborted children's tissue;

- no abortion and donation should be permitted between relatives;

- abortion procedures (e.g., the timing or method of abortion) should not be altered to accommodate the potential use of fetal tissue. (9)

These stipulations and restrictions are intended to prevent the encouragement of abortion (9), since such encouragement could be seen as constituting one form of complicity in abortion. (10) Further, several restrictions are intended to discourage a woman from starting a pregnancy with the sole intent of aborting the fetus to provide therapies for family members, friends, or acquaintances. (9)

On the other hand, some have not seen these restrictions and stipulations as sufficient to prevent complicity in abortion. For example, the Committee for Pro-Life Activities of the National Conference of Catholic Bishops took this position in a statement sent to the NIH Human Fetal Tissue Transplantation Research Panel:

> It may not be wrong in principle for someone unconnected with an abortion to make use of a fetal organ from an unborn child who died as the result of an abortion; but it is difficult to see how this practice can be institutionalized without threatening a morally unacceptable collaboration with the abortion industry. (9)

In defense of using tissue from electively aborted fetuses, an analogy is often drawn with the transplant of organs and tissue from homicide and accident victims:

> Families of murder and accident victims are often asked to donate organs and bodies for research, therapy and education. If they consent, organ procurement agencies retrieve the organs and distribute them to recipients unconnected with organ retrieval. No one would seriously argue that the surgeon who transplants the homicide or accident victim's kidneys, heart, liver or corneas or the recipient who receives it become accomplices in the homicide or accident that made the organs available. Nor is the medical student who uses the cadaver of a murder victim to study anatomy an accomplice in that murder. (9)

However, this analogy has been criticized on the grounds that it ignores the aspect of an "institutional partnership...whereby the bodily remains of abortion victims become a regularly supplied medical commodity." (9) While no one would seriously argue that the transplant surgeon is an accomplice in the homicide or accident that made the organs available, "such a serious argument could be made, however, if the surgeon contracted with the murderer to provide him organs for transplantation, to tell him when and where the organs would be made available, to arrange for the surgeon and his agents to be present to have the organs in "fresh" condition, and to reimburse the murderer for any expenses incurred in making the organs available." (9) And, it is claimed, "these are the types of arrangement that are routinely made to obtain fetal tissue." (9) In other words, it is contended that a more appropriate analogy for the use of tissue from aborted fetuses would be the case of a particular hospital becoming the beneficiary of an organized homicide-system that provides a regular supply of fresh cadavers. (9) And, in such a case, it is argued "one would be justified in raising questions about the moral appropriateness of the hospital's continuing cooperation with the suppliers." (9)

In the debate concerning the use of tissue from aborted fetuses, various analyses have been proposed of what would constitute "complicity" in abortion. (10) One form of complicity would be "causal responsibility for particular abortions"; that is, directly influencing a woman to have an abortion. (10) Women confronted with a problem pregnancy may be ambivalent about having an abortion. (9) It is feared that the good that may come from the use of tissue from aborted fetuses (such as the extraction of stem cells for therapeutic purposes) may serve as a reason or motivation in a woman's mind for having the abortion:

> Indeed, one bioethicist claims that "There's a strong argument that intending to use tissue to relieve someone else's disease is a better ethical act than having an abortion just because you forgot to use a diaphragm." Thus, a powerful human motivation will be thrown into the balance for women considering abortion: concern for others. The decision to abort, once difficult and troubling, becomes, for some, a noble and selfless act of "doing good for humanity." (9)

On the other hand, some have argued that this fear is unfounded. They contend that the "chief motivation for abortion is the desire to avoid the burdens of an unwanted pregnancy" and that even if the donation of fetal tissue makes a woman feel better, this does "not show that tissue donation will lead to a termination decision that would not otherwise have occurred." (9)

Another form of complicity in abortion would consist in "knowingly benefitting from abortions."(10) This is because "a partnership whereby one achieves direct benefit from another person's injurious behavior, after the fact, can place the former in silent but unmistakable alliance with what the latter is doing." (11)

It is certainly true that not all cases of benefiting from immoral actions make one complicitous with the evil acts. (10) For example, "heirs of a murdered relative may benefit financially from the murder, and owners who claim insurance on an abandoned building set on fire may benefit financially from the act of arson" yet "they are not considered complicitous with the murderer or arsonist simply because they benefit from these immoral acts." (10) Further, even persons who repeatedly benefit from immoral acts need not be complicitous in these acts. (10) For example, transplant surgeons and others may benefit from the results of drunken driving, assaults, and murders, but they do not directly intend to benefit from these immoral acts. (10) In sum, it is "the premeditated, intentional seeking of benefit from the wrongdoing of others that may constitute complicity in wrongdoing." (10)

In the case of using tissue from aborted fetuses, a study from the Center for Biomedical Ethics at the University of Minnesota has described an escape route from charges of complicity of this type:

> Researchers and others benefit from the practice of abortion, which, depending on one's point of view, is likely to include at least some immoral abortions. Whether those who benefit from the use of fetal tissue are open to the charge of being complicit with those who engage in immoral abortions by virtue of knowingly benefitting from these abortions, may depend on whether they directly intend to use tissue specifically from fetuses aborted for immoral reasons or whether they merely tolerate that some of the tissue may come from fetuses aborted for immoral reasons. The large differences of opinion regarding which elective abortions are immoral and how much "immoral tissue" may be in the supply of fetal tissue before it is impermissible to use tissue from any electively aborted fetuses, results in different conclusions about when it may be justifiable to charge those who benefit from the use of fetal tissue with complicity due to knowingly benefitting from immoral abortions. (10)

When analyzed, this escape route presupposes that at least some abortions may be morally permissible. If one holds the belief that abortion is always immoral, then one cannot decide to use tissue from aborted fetuses without directly intending to benefit from the wrongdoing of others. Thus, given the aforementioned analysis of complicity with wrongdoing, the belief that abortion is always immoral leads to the conclusion that obtaining stem cells from aborted fetuses involves an unacceptable complicity with abortion. (12)

Ethics of Embryonic Stem Cell Research

There are three possible sources of embryonic stem cells: spare frozen embryos at reproductive clinics, embryos that have been deliberately created for research purposes using sperm and ova, and cloned embryos. All three types of embryos are created in vitro. There are some who do not regard this reproductive technology as ethically permissible. (13) For these individuals, an objection already exists at this level to embryonic stem cell research.

However, the main line of controversy about embryonic stem cell research revolves around the status of the early embryo, which is destroyed in the process of obtaining stem cells. Is this early embryo a human being with a right to life? *Newsweek* magazine captured the essence of this controversy in a subtitle below a picture of the early embryo: "What is the *value* of this clump of cells? Another *human* or a new hope for the diseased and dying?" (14)

Three views have emerged on the standing of the early embryo from an ethical point of view. One view accords full human status and rights to the early embryo. A second view regards it as no different than any other human tissue. A third view, attempting to delineate a middle ground, accords the embryo greater respect than is afforded other human tissue but does not grant it full personal status. (15)

The third position has been taken by the Ethics Advisory Board for Geron, a bio-pharmaceutical company working with embryonic stem cells. Specifically, this Ethics Advisory Board has adopted a developmental view of human personhood and moral status: as the conceptus develops from blastocyst to fetus and beyond, so too does its moral status grow. (16) The Board affirms the principle of respect for human life, but their developmental view has the consequence that this principle entails different obligations at different developmental stages. As interpreted by this Board, "early embryonic tissue is respected by ensuring that it is used with care only in research that incorporates substantive values such as reduction of human suffering." (16) And, according to this Board, the potential of human embryonic stem cell research "to contribute to fundamental knowledge of human development and to medical and pharmaceutical interventions to alleviate suffering" does "provide such substantive values...." (16)

On the other hand, it is pointed out that the genetic material for a new being—technically, its "genome"—is put together at fertilization. This set of genes determines that it will develop as human (rather than another sort of plant or animal) and influences at least some of its individual traits. (13, 17) Further, fertilization represents the beginning of a continuous process of development that will eventually result in the birth of a child. These considerations are taken as reasons for picking fertilization as the beginning of a human life.

Some have recently challenged these arguments on biological grounds. One line of objection is based on the view that speaking of a human being in existence requires *individuality* in the entity. However, the early embryo can split to form identical twins (or triplets or more), allegedly providing evidence that the early embryo is not yet one human being, but in effect a community of possibly different individuals. (4) Another argument proposed against human individuality at this stage of development is the fact that separate and genetically distinct embryos—which might have gone on to become fraternal twins—sometimes fuse during early development to form a single human being. Second, the phenomenon of natural wastage is cited, that is, the failure of early embryos to implant in a woman's uterus in order to continue their development. Such embryos are simply discharged from the woman's body. Although estimates of the rate of natural wastage vary, some claim that between two-thirds and three-quarters of all fertilized ova do not go on to implant in the womb. (4) Hence, the question is raised: "In view of this high rate of embryonic loss, do we truly want to bestow much moral significance on an entity with which nature is so wasteful?" (4)

Those who hold the view that a human life, properly speaking, begins at fertilization have attempted to refute the alleged implications of the biological phenomena in question. For example, in response to natural wastage, it has been pointed out that, historically, at least 50 percent of all infants died in infancy, yet this mortality rate does not make us think that these infants were not fully human. (18, 19) Further, since the process of syngamy (the fusion of the nuclei of the ovum and sperm into the single nucleus of the zygote) can fail to complete, it has been speculated "many of these imperfectly fertilized ova were never truly human organisms." (18) With respect to the phenomenon of twinning, it is contended that the "embryological evidence suggests not that the original organism splits, but that it remains itself but loses one or more cells that become the twin." (18) Concomitantly, it is argued that "the fact that a group of cells is able after separation to develop independently into a second individuated organism in no way refutes the prior existence of an individuated organism...." (18)

Before concluding this discussion of the ethics of embryonic stem cell research, there is another issue in this debate that deserves attention. Specifically, some argue that there is a difference between deliberately creating embryos to obtain stem cells and obtaining them from spare frozen embryos remaining at reproductive clinics. In the latter case, the embryos may eventually be destroyed anyway. So the argument is made that it would be preferable to use them for the greater good of research that has the potential to save and improve other human lives. (20)

In rebuttal of this line of argument, it has been pointed out that "we do not kill terminally ill patients for their organs, although they will die soon anyway, or even harvest vital organs from death row prisoners, although they will be put to death soon anyway." (21) Further, it has been pointed out that "Federal law prohibits federally funded researchers from doing any harm to an unborn child slated for abortion, though that child will soon be discarded anyway (see 42 USC 289g)." (21)

Federal Funding for Embryonic Stem Cell Research

On August 9, 2001, President George W. Bush announced a policy that federal funds may be used only for research on some sixty stem cell lines already in existence "where the life-and-death decision has already been made." (20) According to President Bush, "This allows us to explore the promise and potential of stem cell research without crossing a fundamental moral line by providing taxpayer funding that would sanction or encourage further destruction of human embryos that have at least the potential for life." (20)

In particular, Bush's policy allows federal funds to be used only for research on then-existing stem cell lines that were derived with the informed consent of the donors, from excess embryos created solely for reproductive purposes, and without any financial inducements to the donors. No federal funds may be used for the derivation of stem cell lines coming from newly destroyed embryos, the creation of any human embryos for research purposes, or the cloning of human embryos for any purpose. (22) It should be noted that this policy applies only to federally funded research, and does not impact the work of privately financed biopharmaceutical companies.

Among those regarded as pro-life, there has been a mixed reaction to the position taken by President Bush. David N. O'Steen, executive director of the National Right to Life Committee, praised Bush's decision:

The substantive and symbolic importance of the president's decision for the pro-life movement should not be underestimated. ...The National Right to Life Committee commends Bush's decision to prevent the federal government from becoming involved in research that would require the destruction of human embryos. In so doing, the president acted to save the lives that he could. (23)

On the other hand, Reverend Michael Place, President and CEO of the Catholic Health Association of the United States, saw Bush's position as flawed:

> ...what could appear as a carefully nuanced solution to a complex issue— utilizing the already existing cultured stem cell lines—itself raises significant moral concerns for our society. Because these cell lines resulted from the destruction of human embryonic life, their origin is morally reprehensible. The continued use of these cultured stem cell lines by scientists involves complicity in the destruction of embryonic human life. (24)

In order to understand Place's position, it is necessary to recognize the framework within which his statement is made. First, his position assumes that it is ethically wrong to destroy an early embryo. Second, it assumes an understanding of complicity discussed earlier; namely, that the premeditated, intentional seeking of benefit from the wrongdoing of others makes one complicitous with that wrongdoing. (10)

A further objection has been raised to Bush's position based on the canons of research ethics. This is the contention that "the federal government, for the first time in history, will support research that relies on the destruction of some defenseless human beings for the possible benefit to others." (25) Bush's policy is seen as "treating some human lives as nothing more than objects to be manipulated and destroyed for research purposes." (25) This line of objection again presupposes a view of the early embryo as having the status and rights of a human being. This brings us back to what is a central issue in the ethical debate about embryonic stem cell research.

FOR GROUP DISCUSSION

1. Embryonic stem cell research is an ethical issue that has spilled over into the arena of public policy. During a debate on embryonic stem cell research in the U.S. House of Representatives, one House member made the following comment in support of such research: "We must not say to millions of sick and injured human beings, 'go ahead and die, stay paralyzed, because we believe the blastocyst, the clump of cells, is more important than you are.' ...It is a sentence of death to millions of Americans." (2) What is your reaction to this comment?

2. Another member of Congress made this comment in support of embryonic stem cell research: "If your religious beliefs will not allow you to accept a cure for your child's cancer, so be it. But do not expect the rest of America to let their loved ones suffer without cure." (2) What is your reaction to this comment?

3. In spite of some opposition, embryonic stem cell research may well go forward. Suppose that, in our case study, Martha learns that the tissue to be implanted into her father was developed from embryonic stem cells and that she personally considers embryonic stem cell research to be morally wrong. Given that Martha had no part in how the therapy was developed and given its potential for significant benefit for her father, do you think it is ethically permissible for Martha to agree to the use of this therapy even though she regards the way it was developed as morally wrong?

NOTES

1. National Institutes of Health, *Stem Cells: Scientific Progress and Future Research* (July 2001). http://www.nih.gov/news/stemcell

2. United States Conference of Catholic Bishops, Secretariat for Pro-Life Activities, "The Human Embryo as Research Commodity," *Life Insight* 12/4 (Aug.-Sept. 2001).

3. National Institutes of Health, *Stem Cells: A Primer* (May 2000). http://www.nih.gov/news/stemcell

4. Ronald M. Green, *The Human Embryo Research Debates* (New York: Oxford, 2001).

5. News@UW-Madison, "Wisconsin scientists culture elusive embryonic stem cells," Nov. 5, 1998. http://www.news.wisc.edu/packages/stemcells

6. Advanced Cell Technology, "Human Therapeutic Cloning Program." http://www.advancedcell.com

7. CNN, "Researchers isolate human stem cells in the lab," Nov. 5, 1998. http://www.cnn.com/HEALTH/9811/05/stemcell.discovery

8. Do No Harm—The Coalition of Americans for Research Ethics. http://www.stemcellresearch.org

9. Human Fetal Tissue Transplantation Research Panel, National Institutes of Health, *Report of the Human Fetal Tissue Transplantation Research Panel*, 2 vols. (Springfield, VA: U.S. Department of Commerce, National Technical Information Service, 1988).

10. Dorothy E. Vawter et al., *The Use of Human Fetal Tissue: Scientific, Ethical, and Policy Concerns* (Minneapolis, MN: Center for Biomedical Ethics, University of Minnesota, 1990).

11. James Tunstead Burtchaell, "University Policy on Experimental Use of Aborted Fetal Tissue," *IRB: A Review of Human Subjects Research* 10/4 (July/August 1988): 7-11.

12. This discussion of the ethics of using tissue from aborted fetuses is excerpted and adapted from *Church Teaching on Health Care Ethics A Handbook of Policies for the Archdiocese of Dubuque* (Dubuque, IA: Archdiocese of Dubuque, 1988 -).

13. Congregation for the Doctrine of the Faith, *Instruction on Respect for Human Life in its Origin and On the Dignity of Procreation* (Washington, DC: United States Catholic Conference, 1987).

14. Kenneth L. Woodward, "A Question of Life or Death," *Newsweek* (July 9, 2001): 31.

15. Thomas A. Shannon and Lisa Sowle Cahill, *Religion and Artificial Reproduction* (New York: Crossroad, 1988).

16. Geron Ethics Advisory Board, "Research with Human Embryonic Stem Cells: Ethical Considerations," *Hastings Center Report* 29 (1999): 31-36.

17. John T. Noonan, Jr., *The Morality of Abortion: Legal and Historical Perspectives* (Cambridge, MA: Harvard University Press, 1970).

18. Benedict M. Ashley, OP and Kevin D. O'Rourke, OP, *Health Care Ethics A Theological Analysis*, 4th ed. (Washington, DC: Georgetown University Press, 1997).

19. John Mahoney, *Bioethics and Belief* (London: Sheed and Ward, 1984).

20. The Washington Post, "Bush Announces Position on Stem Cell Research." http://www.washingtonpost.com/wp-srv/onpolitics/transcripts/bushtext_080901.htm

21. Richard Doerflinger, *Testimony at Congressional Hearings on Embryo Stem Cell Research*, July 18, 2001. http://www.nccbuscc.org/comm/commcur.htm

22. Office of the Press Secretary, The White House, "Fact Sheet Embryonic Stem Cell Research," August 9, 2001. http://www.whitehouse.gov/news/releases/2001/08/print/20010809-1.html

23. "Did Bush Get It Right on Stem Cells?" *National Catholic Register* 77/35 (Sept. 2-8, 2001) at 4.

24. Catholic Health Association of the United States, News Release, August 9, 2001.

25. Bishop Joseph A. Fiorenza, " Catholic Bishops Criticize Bush Policy on Embryo Research" (August 9, 2001). http://www.nccbuscc.org/comm/archives/2001/01-142.htm

FOR FURTHER STUDY

- Suzanne Holland and Karen Lebacqz (eds.), *Human Embryonic Stem Cell Debate: Science, Ethics, and Public Policy* (Cambridge: MIT Press, 2001).

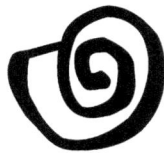

Appendix

Ethical Theory

Most books about health care ethics begin with a discussion of ethical principles and theories, which are later applied to concrete problems in health care. In contrast, this book deals with ethics contextually, introducing ethical principles and theories as they naturally arise in the course of discussing concrete ethical dilemmas.

This appendix will give a more systematic exposition of the ethical principles and theories introduced in the various chapters. Ethical theories will be explained in greater detail. It will be shown how various principles are related to each other. Finally, some criticisms of these principles and theories will be discussed.

Four Basic Principles of Health Care Ethics

In *Principles of Biomedical Ethics*, a work that has now become a classic of health care ethics, Tom L. Beauchamp and James F. Childress reduce all of health care ethics to four basic principles: autonomy, beneficence, nonmaleficence, and justice. (1) These principles are sometimes referred to as the "Georgetown mantra" because of the association of the philosophers who developed them with the Kennedy Institute of Ethics at Georgetown University. (1, 2) We have explained these principles in the following way:

> *Autonomy:* self-determination; the right of an individual to make the final decision in matters pertaining to his or her own life and health care.
>
> *Beneficence:* the duty of a health care worker to promote the health and well-being of patients and residents.
>
> *Nonmaleficence:* the duty of a health care worker to prevent harm from coming to patients and residents.
>
> *Justice:* an ethical principle concerning fairness in the distribution of benefits, burdens and resources.

On this scheme of doing ethics, ethical dilemmas can be generated when more than one of these principles is applicable to a situation and the principles conflict in directing what course of action ought to be taken. For example, suppose that a nursing home resident who is dying says that she wants "everything done," including transfer to the intensive care unit (ICU) of the local hospital. Let us further suppose that her physician believes that ICU care would prolong her life for a few days at the most, and that he fears that her presence in the ICU might take a bed away from an emergency case coming into the hospital whose recovery would be greatly helped by ICU care. This case involves a conflict between individual autonomy and justice in the allocation of health care resources. Autonomy directs that the resident should be placed in the ICU. Justice, on the other hand, mandates that the resources of the ICU be reserved for someone who can genuinely benefit from them and not be "wasted" on this particular nursing home resident. In such cases of conflict, a judgment must be made as to which principle is more important. The weightier principle then tells us the right thing to do. (2)

As indicated by the number of times it is mentioned in this text, autonomy has come to occupy a central place in contemporary health care ethics. Indeed, autonomy provides the grounding for several other principles in health care ethics. The principle of substituted judgment directs a proxy decision maker to make treatment decisions in accord with the values and wishes of the resident. In this respect, it represents an extension of autonomy (self-determination) to situations in which the resident is no longer capable of making treatment decisions directly. Further, procedures for obtaining the free and informed consent of the resident for participation in research projects respect the resident's right to direct the course of his or her own life.

The emphasis currently being placed on autonomy is, at least in part, a reaction to the paternalistic way in which medicine was practiced at one time. The physician was the one who made treatment decisions, and the resident and family members tended to go along with what the physician said without raising questions. The emphasis on autonomy may also reflect the American emphasis on individualism. (2, 3)

While no one is advocating a return to physician paternalism, some concern is now being raised that the pendulum has swung too far in the other direction. There is concern that autonomy has gone too far and that some limits on it are in order. For example, some are arguing that a patient or resident should not be entitled to receive futile medical treatments and that health care providers have the right to override the patient's or resident's wishes when futile treatments are wanted. (4) Others offer a more radical criticism of the very concept of autonomy, maintaining that a focus on the patient or resident alone is misguided. (2)

The Ethics of Care

Out of feminist work in ethics has come the *ethics of care*. This approach to ethics has been described in the following way:

> ...[G]irls, being brought up by mothers, identify with them, while males must define themselves through separation from their mothers. ...Thus while masculinity is defined by separation and threatened by intimacy, femininity is defined through attachment and threatened by separation; girls come to understand themselves as imbedded within a network of personal relationships... (5)

> The feminine voice in ethics attends to the particular other, thinks in terms of responsibilities to care for others, is sensitive to our interconnectedness, and strives to preserve relationships. It contrasts with the masculine voice, which speaks in terms of justice and rights, stresses consistency and prin-

ciples, and emphasizes the autonomy of the individual and impartiality in one's dealings with others. (5)

This feminist approach to ethics is "frequently described in terms of webs or networks" (2) and emphasizes "relationships and connections" rather than "isolated individuals." (2) The ethics of care "focuses on a set of character traits that people all deeply value in close personal relationships: sympathy, compassion, fidelity, love, friendship, and the like." (6)

It has been claimed that the ethics of care is already part of the way we naturally reason in health care ethics:

> Looking at ethics committees, Sichel argues that a feminist ethics of caring is often part of the ethics committee's deliberations. She uses as an example the case of an incompetent elderly patient whose wishes are known but whose children disagree about what course to follow. She accurately notes that, although the committee will support following the patient's wishes, it will go to considerable lengths and spend considerable time in an attempt to obtain consensus about this course from all the children, believing that it has a duty to care about the family as well as the patient. It would appear that if the patient's wishes were the only important factor, the course of action desired by the patient should be followed immediately, rather than after the children have been persuaded to agree. (2)

In sum, rather than focusing exclusively on what the patient or resident wants (the principle of autonomy), the ethics of care directs us to take into account all the players in an ethical dilemma in working through it.

Religious Contributions to Health Care Ethics

Within the Catholic Church there is a long history of theological work in health care ethics. (7) Two ethical principles discussed in this text have come out of this tradition; namely, the principle of weighing benefits and burdens and the principle of double effect. Natural law ethics, discussed in conjunction with euthanasia and assisted suicide, is also associated with the Catholic tradition.

Historically, Catholic ethicists drew a distinction between *ordinary* and *extraordinary* treatments, and used the principle that ordinary treatments must always be provided, whereas the use of extraordinary treatments is not obligatory. (7) Even today, some people still talk about this distinction and principle when making decisions about life-sustaining treatments.

However, as noted by the President's Commission for the Study of Ethical Problems in Medicine and Biomedical and Behavioral Research, there are problems with this distinction. For one thing, different meanings came to be attached to the terms "ordinary" and "extraordinary." Some interpreted it as a distinction between "common" and "unusual" care whereas others saw it as distinguishing care that is "simple" from care that is "complex" or "elaborate" or "artificial." Furthermore, these different interpretations could yield different judgments about whether a particular treatment is ordinary or extraordinary and should be provided or forgone. For example, resuscitation is a commonly used procedure, which would make it an "ordinary" treatment on the first interpretation. On the other hand, the physical, chemical, and electrical means used in resuscitation attempts can be considered technologically complex, making resuscitation an "extraordinary" means on the second interpretation of the term. (8)

The *Declaration on Euthanasia*, issued in 1980 by the Vatican Congregation for the Doctrine of the Faith, explicitly moved away from the ordinary/extraordinary terminology to speak in terms of *proportionate* and *disproportionate* means. (9) The latter distinction is now commonly interpreted in terms of a consideration of *benefits and burdens*. This evolution of terminology is made explicit in the 1994 revision of the *Ethical and Religious Directives for Catholic Health Care Services*:

> A person has a moral obligation to use ordinary or proportionate means of preserving his or her life. Proportionate means are those that in the judgment of the patient offer a reasonable hope of benefit and do not entail an excessive burden or impose excessive expense on the family or community. (10)

> A person may forgo extraordinary or disproportionate means of preserving life. Disproportionate means are those that in the patient's judgment do not offer a reasonable hope of benefit or entail an excessive burden, or impose excessive expense on the family or the community. (10)

The benefits and burdens principle does not represent a completely new moral criterion for the use of life-sustaining treatments. Rather, it is an attempt to bring about greater clarity and precision by focusing on one of the traditional interpretations of the ordinary/extraordinary distinction. (8) For present purposes, what is significant is that the principle of weighing benefits and burdens has now become the accepted standard for making decisions about life-sustaining treatments in health care ethics generally. (8, 11)

Natural law ethics is associated with the Catholic moral tradition. However, the idea of a natural law goes back to Greek and Roman legal thought, where this idea is found among Stoics and in the writings of Cicero. Natural law theory flourished in the high and late Middle Ages. In this period the classic statement of natural law theory was given by Thomas Aquinas, but many other philosophers and theologians held it as well. (12) Natural law theory continued into the early Modern period, being found in the writings of such philosophers as Thomas Hobbes (13) and John Locke. (14) Among all the theories that go under the name of natural law, there is a common core of beliefs that the basic principles of morals and legislation are, in some sense or other, objective, accessible to reason, and based on human nature. (12)

In its classic form as presented by Aquinas, natural law ethics holds that what is in accord with human nature is to be considered right, and what goes against human nature is to be considered wrong. More exactly, human nature has certain properties. These properties entail that a human being ought to do acts a, b, and c and ought not to do acts x, y, and z. (12)

For example, human beings have a natural inclination to self-preservation. What is in accord with self-preservation is right. Thus, it is right to exercise regularly in order to keep in shape physically since this promotes self-preservation. On the other hand, assisted suicide and euthanasia go against the natural inclination to self-preservation, and hence are wrong actions.

Natural law has recently been used by the Catholic Church in evaluating technologies of assisted reproduction. For example, the Catholic Church has used natural law reasoning to rule out the use of in vitro fertilization. What occurs naturally is that the act of intercourse has two functions: an expression of love between two people and the conception of a child. It is *unnatural* to separate the conception of a child from intercourse, but by fertilizing an ovum in a dish in a laboratory, this is precisely what in vitro fertilization does. Hence, according to natural law ethics, in vitro fertilization is to be judged morally impermissible. (15)

A point presented in favor of natural law theory is that it provides a basis from which to address all people, without regard to their particular religious tradition. (16) This is so because it bases right and wrong on a human nature common to all people. On the other hand, exactly what is human nature? Can we spell out precisely what properties it includes?

It should also be noted that the principle of double effect has come out of the natural law tradition. The one mentioned in this text is the principle of double effect. Basically, this principle justifies taking a course of action that has two types of effects: one effect is perfectly good and is really wanted while the other one is bad and is not wanted but may accompany the first. (17) Within the Catholic tradition, the principle of double effect has traditionally been used to justify the removal of a cancerous uterus when a woman is pregnant. The desired effect is the removal of a diseased organ, which is a perfectly legitimate aim. In the case of pregnancy, however, removing the cancerous uterus will also mean the death of the fetus. The woman who is pregnant may not want to lose the child she is carrying, but this will be an unavoidable effect of removing the diseased organ. (17)

In its fully developed form, the principle of double effect includes stipulations such as that the act itself must be morally good or neutral, that only the good consequences of the act must be intended, that the good effect must not be produced by means of the evil effect, and that there must be some weighty reason for permitting the evil. (8) For example, the act of removing a diseased organ, such as a cancerous uterus, is at least morally neutral and very possibly can be considered a morally good action. If a woman feels a loss because of the death of her child, it is clear that it is only the good consequence of removing a diseased organ that is intended by her, not the evil effect of the death of the child. If the cancerous uterus were removed with the fetus in it (rather than the fetus being killed before the removal of the uterus), then the evil effect of the death of the child would not be the means of achieving the good effect. Finally, saving the life of the woman by removing a cancerous organ is certainly a weighty reason for permitting the evil of the death of her fetus.

As noted in the discussion of pain management, the principle of double effect has been used to justify the administration of pain medication that may have a side effect of hastening death. (8) While almost everyone would agree that this course of action is morally permissible, not everyone would accept the principle of double effect as an appropriate justification for this action. This principle holds that death cannot be used as the means of relieving suffering but that it can be accepted as merely a foreseeable consequence of relieving suffering. Some have taken issue with this distinction, maintaining that "people are equally responsible for all of the foreseeable effects of their actions." (8) They see the real moral issue as "whether or not the decision makers have considered the full range of foreseeable effects, have knowingly accepted whatever risk of death is entailed, and have found the risk to be justified in light of the paucity and undesirability of other options." (8)

Consequentialist vs. Nonconsequentialist Theories

In this book, both utilitarianism and Kantian ethics have been mentioned. These two ethical systems represent different types of ethical theory. Utilitarianism is a *consequentialist* ethical theory—a theory that judges rightness and wrongness on the basis of the consequences of action. Kantian ethics is one example of a *nonconsequentialist* (or *deontological*) theory. This type of theory maintains either that factors entirely apart from consequences determine the rightness or wrongness of action, or that factors in addition to consequences are relevant.

Historically, utilitarianism was formulated by two British philosophers, Jeremy Bentham (1748-1832) and John Stuart Mill (1806-1873). It is commonly known as the philosophy of "the greatest good for the greatest number." Utilitarianism requires us to consider consequences for everyone to be affected by a course of action. In this respect it differs from the consequentialist theory of ethical egoism, which directs us to consider only the consequences of an action for oneself.

Consider reasons offered for and against surrogate motherhood. On the one hand, surrogacy provides a wanted child to an infertile couple. It allows the child to be biologically related to the father. And, given the shortage of children available for adoption, it can provide an infertile couple with a child more quickly. On the other hand, the surrogate mother can become attached to the child she is carrying and find giving up the child to be emotionally traumatic. Indeed, she may decide she wants to keep the child, with ensuing court battles. If the surrogate is willing to give up the child but is herself married and has her own children, these children may experience a sense of loss at being deprived of a sibling. If the child born in a surrogacy arrangement turns out to be mentally or physically handicapped, neither the surrogate mother nor the contracting couple may want the child, and the child may end up in a state institution. (18, 19, 20)

When analyzed, all the aforementioned reasons for and against surrogacy represent positive and negative consequences of surrogate motherhood. Further, consequences are discussed for a variety of people impacted by the surrogate motherhood arrangement: the infertile couple, the woman who serves as a surrogate mother, children of the surrogate mother, the child born through the surrogacy arrangement, and society at large. Thus, the above paragraph represents a utilitarian way of thinking about the moral permissibility of surrogate motherhood.

Since the time of Bentham and Mill, several different types of utilitarianism have been formulated. Perhaps the simplest form of utilitarianism is *act-utilitarianism*, which focuses on particular courses of action. This theory analyzes rightness of action in the following way:

> Act A is right when, from among the courses of action which could be taken in the situation, act A is the one which will have the best consequences overall when everyone to be affected by the action is taken into account.

How would this principle be used by staff of a long-term care facility in determining whether a male resident who is currently living with his wife in the general health care unit should be transferred to the facility's special dementia unit? These are the steps they would follow:

> (1) They determine the courses of action which can be taken, namely, allow the resident to remain in the general health care unit with his wife or transfer the resident to the special dementia unit.
>
> (2) For each of these courses of action, they figure out the possible consequences of that course of action. They figure out the possible consequences of allowing the resident to remain in his present living arrangement, and the possible consequences of transferring him to the special dementia unit. Consequences are considered for everyone who will be affected by the action (e.g., the resident himself, the resident's wife, other residents of the facility, the facility's staff), and long-range as well as immediate consequences are taken into account.
>
> (3) Since some of the consequences listed are likely to be "good" or "positive" while others are likely to be "bad" or "negative," the positive and negative consequences are weighed against each other for each course of action to determine an overall value for that course of action.
>
> (4) The overall values of the courses of action are compared. In this case, the overall value of allowing the resident to remain in his present room with his wife versus the overall value of transferring him to the special dementia unit.
>
> (5) The course of action which overall has the best consequences is the right one to perform.

Other types of utilitarianism, rather than focusing on particular actions, consider the consequences of adopting a certain set of rules (21) or the consequences of people generally performing a certain type of action. (22) Some versions of utilitarianism (such as that first formulated by Bentham and Mill) judge consequences hedonistically, in terms of the pleasure and pain produced. (23, 24) On the other hand, a recent variant of utilitarianism makes such judgments in terms of people's actual preferences. (21)

For the utilitarian, no action is intrinsically right or wrong. Rightness and wrongness are determined entirely by consequences. Consider, for example, the issue of confidentiality discussed in this book. According to the utilitarian, "if violating confidentiality seems necessary to produce a state of affairs in which happiness is increased, then the violation is justified." (25) This might occur, for instance, "when someone's life is in danger or someone is being tried for a serious crime and the testimony of a physician is needed to help establish her innocence." (25)

Utilitarianism requires us to consider consequences of actions not only for ourselves, but for everyone who will be affected by what we do. In this regard, John Stuart Mill commended utilitarianism as embodying the Christian spirit:

> ...the happiness which forms the utilitarian standard of what is right in conduct is not the agent's own happiness but that of all concerned. As between his own happiness and that of others, utilitarianism requires him to be as strictly impartial as a disinterested and benevolent spectator. In the golden rule of Jesus of Nazareth, we read the complete spirit of the ethics of utility. "To do as you would be done by," and "to love your neighbor as yourself," constitute the ideal perfection of utilitarian morality. (24)

As another point in favor of utilitarianism, it is claimed that utilitarianism reflects our ordinary ethical thinking. It is claimed that we ordinarily look at consequences of actions in deciding what ought to be done. Some are attracted to utilitarianism because it forces us to take time to figure out and consider the consequences of our actions. Utilitarianism forces us to be reflective about ethical decisions rather than making them quickly on the basis of initial reactions.

On the other hand, there are some practical difficulties with applying utilitarianism. Do we always have the time to consider all the possible consequences of our actions before a choice must be made? Just consider the case of an emergency room physician who has to decide whether to use a new drug on a patient brought in for a heart attack. Can we really determine what all the consequences of our actions may be in the long run? Our actions can have unforeseeable ripple effects. For example, marriage partners often meet in college settings. Whom an individual marries will determine much about the course of that person's life, for example, number of children, the particular children he or she has, home environment, geographical mobility, levels of personal satisfaction and happiness. But can anyone foresee all these possible consequences when choosing which college to attend?

Another objection against utilitarianism is an intuitive feeling that factors other than consequences do count in making ethical judgments. For example, the very fact that a promise has been made should count for something, quite apart from the consequences of keeping or breaking the promise. Or again, we believe that it is simply unjust to punish an innocent person, even if punishing him in the circumstances might have good consequences overall. (26)

An ethical theory that makes judgments apart from the consequences of actions is that of Immanuel Kant (1724-1804). Kant named his ethical theory the *categorical imperative*. He gave different formulations of the categorical imperative, stating his fundamental moral principle in different ways. The two most famous formulations are the *universal law* formula, and the *end in itself* formula. It is the second formulation of the categorical imperative that has been used in this text.

Kant stated the end in itself formula in this way: "So act as to treat humanity, whether in thine own person or in that of any other, in every case as an end withal, never as a means only... " (27) Here is an explanation of what he means:

> According to this formulation, rational creatures should always treat other rational creatures as ends in themselves and never as only means to ends. This formulation underscores Kant's belief that every human being has an inherent worth resulting from the sheer possession of rationality. We must always act in a way that respects this humanity in others and in ourselves. (28)

According to Kant, we act wrongly if we merely "use" another person to get something we want. We act rightly only if we treat human beings, both other people and ourselves, as beings having intrinsic worth.

For example, some of the arguments offered against the ethical permissibility of surrogate motherhood are applications of this Kantian moral principle:

> This makes it appear that surrogacy is unethical because of the type of practice it is, namely, a form of exploitation. According to one writer: "When a woman provides womb service, the feminist issue surfaces. Women object to being baby factories or sex objects because it offends their human dignity." And further: "This is going to end up as the final exploitation of women. It is always going to be poor women who have the babies and rich women who get them."
>
> ...to treat one's body as a mere means to the ends of others is degrading. It could be viewed as a violation of Kant's supreme moral principle, the categorical imperative, which prohibits treating persons merely as a means. (29)

Thus both utilitarians and Kantians have arguments pertaining to surrogate motherhood, but their arguments are of different types.

It is very important to recognize that utilitarians and Kantians can come to different conclusions about the right thing to do in a particular case. Suppose, for example, that an elderly woman is dying of cancer and that all known treatments have failed to help her. Her physicians suggest use of an experimental drug. The physicians do not believe that the drug will help this woman. In fact, they candidly tell her that she is likely to suffer from fever and vomiting if she takes the drug (which will increase her suffering as she dies). However, if she does take the drug, the physicians will gain information about how elderly cancer patients tolerate it. This information will be valuable in using the drug with other older cancer patients who may be helped by it. (30) A Kantian would be against giving the woman the experimental drug because she would simply be used to gain knowledge for the benefit of other people. A utilitarian, on the other hand, would favor the administration of the experimental drug because of the good consequences overall. While the woman will suffer, the negative value of her suffering will be outweighed by the good consequences for other people.

This case illustrates another objection which has been brought against utilitarianism, namely, that it can sacrifice the individual for the sake of the group. (26) On the other hand, Kant's end in itself formula of the categorical imperative has been criticized on the grounds that "it is not always clear when people are being treated as ends and when as means." (28) For example, Kant judged prostitution to be immoral "because, by selling their sexual services, prostitutes allow themselves to be treated as means." (28) However, there is a sense in which anyone who works for a wage also sells his or her services. (28) So "does that mean that we are all being treated immorally, because our employers are presumably hiring us as a means to advance their own ends?" (28) This question might be answered negatively on the grounds that we have freely agreed to do the work. But then the same is true of the prostitute. (28)

Ethical Relativism

The position known as *ethical relativism* denies that there is a single, objectively true moral standard that is valid for everyone everywhere. The relativist maintains that what is right and wrong varies among different cultures and societies. Thus, according to the relativist, euthanasia and assisted suicide may be ethically right in one culture but wrong in another. In making this claim, the relativist is not speaking merely of what people may think is right or wrong, because people can make mistakes in their moral judgments. Rather, the relativist is asserting that what in fact is right or wrong varies among different cultures and societies.

Ethical relativism is *not* itself an ethical theory or principle. Rather, it makes a claim that no ethical theory or principle holds good for everyone everywhere. According to the relativist, utilitarianism may be an appropriate ethical theory for one society but not for another. The principle of autonomy may be right for North Americans but not for Asians.

Prima facie, ethical relativism may seem a very attractive position. For one thing, it seems to take into account the obvious, undeniable fact that different groups of people do differ in their moral judgments. Usury (taking interest on money) was considered wrong in the Old Testament, but today most persons practicing a religion consider this practice to be morally acceptable. Mormons consider it morally permissible for a man to have multiple wives at the same time (polygamy); other Church denominations do not. Hindus consider it wrong to kill and eat a cow, whereas the production of beef for food is a major industry in the United States. Subcultures within a society can also make radically different moral judgments. Just consider the debates over abortion and homosexuality in the United States!

The West has sometimes suffered from *ethnocentrism*, that is, the belief that its culture is inherently superior to other cultures. Such a view has been condemned "as a variety of prejudice tantamount to racism and sexism." A reaction to ethnocentrism is a movement "not to judge others but to be tolerant of diversity." Ethical relativism seems to fit with such an "attitude of tolerance toward other cultures." (31) This is another argument in favor of it.

Some philosophers, however, have argued that ethical relativism has implications that go against common sense and common practice. These unacceptable implications are reasons for judging ethical relativism to be incorrect.

For one thing, ethical relativism prevents us from ever criticizing the practices of another society as evil:

> Suppose a society waged war on its neighbors for the purpose of taking slaves. Or suppose a society was violently anti-Semitic, and its leaders set out to destroy the Jews. Cultural Relativism would preclude us from saying that either of these practices was wrong. We would not even be able to say that a society tolerant of Jews is *better* than the anti-Semitic society, for that would imply some sort of transcultural standard of comparison. The failure to condemn *these* practices does not seem "enlightened"; on the contrary, slavery and anti-Semitism seem wrong *wherever* they occur. Nevertheless, if we took Cultural Relativism seriously, we would have to admit that these social practices also are immune from criticism. (32)

These societal practices would be immune from criticism precisely because what is right and wrong is determined by the particular society.

Moreover, ethical relativism destroys our notion of social reform. For relativism "seems to entail that reformers are always (morally) wrong, because they go against the cultural tide." (31) However, "we normally feel just the opposite: that the reformer is the courageous innovator who is right, who has the truth, against the mindless majority." (31)

Further, ethical relativism destroys the notion of moral progress. This point can be illustrated by the changing status of women in society:

> Usually, we think that at least some changes in our society have been for the better. ...Throughout most of Western history the place of women in society was very narrowly circumscribed. They could not own property; they could not vote or hold political office; with a few exceptions, they were not permitted to have paying jobs; and generally they were under the almost absolute control of their husbands. Recently much of this has changed, and most people think of it as progress.
>
> If Cultural Relativism is correct, can we legitimately think of this as progress? Progress means replacing a way of doing things with a *better* way. But by what standard do we judge the new ways as better? If the old ways were in accordance with the social standards of their time, then Cultural Relativism would say it is a mistake to judge them by the standards of a different time. Eighteenth-century society was, in effect, a

different society from the one we have now. To say that we have made progress implies a judgment that present-day society is better, and that is just the sort of transcultural judgment that, according to Cultural Relativism, is impermissible. (32)

However, it does make sense to think that our society has made some moral progress. Because ethical relativism "says that these judgments make no sense," so the argument goes, "it cannot be right." (32)

According to ethical relativism, right and wrong are determined by a culture or society. This contention entails yet another problem because "one person may belong to several societies (subcultures) with different value emphases and arrangements of principles." (31) For example, "if Mary is a U.S. citizen and a member of the Roman Catholic Church, she is wrong (as a Catholic) if she chooses to have an abortion and not wrong (as a U.S. citizen) if she acts against the teaching of the Church on abortion." (31) According to relativism, just what is the ethically right thing for Mary to do?

If ethical relativism is flawed and there are universal ethical standards, how does one account for the diversity of ethical judgments actually found in our world? Here is one explanation:

> Consider a culture in which people believe it is wrong to eat cows. This may even be a poor culture, in which there is not enough food; still, the cows are not to be touched. Such a society would *appear* to have values very different from our own. But does it? We have not yet asked why these people will not eat cows. Suppose it is because they believe that after death the souls of humans inhabit the bodies of animals, especially cows, so that a cow may be someone's grandmother. Now do we want to say that their values are different from ours? No, the difference lies elsewhere. The difference is in our belief systems, not in our values. We agree that we shouldn't eat Grandma; we simply disagree about whether the cow is (or could be) Grandma. (32)

In other words, opponents of ethical relativism claim that different cultures and societies may share the same basic ethical principles and values but put these principles and values into practice in different ways because of different factual beliefs. Or the same principles and values may be put into practice in different ways because of different circumstances. For example, it has been suggested that Eskimos kill perfectly normal infants *not* because they have less affection for their children or less respect for human life than we do, but for reasons having to do with their life-style and survival. Eskimo mothers will nurse their children for four years, which places limits on the number of infants that one mother can sustain. In addition, Eskimos are nomadic since they are unable to farm, and a mother can carry only one baby as she travels. (32)

If flaws are pointed out in ethical relativism, can anything be said positively in favor of ethical absolutism, the position that there are moral standards that hold true for everyone everywhere? It has been argued "there are some moral rules that all societies will have in common, because those rules are necessary for society to exist." (32)

A prohibition against lying is given as one example:

> Imagine what it would be like for a society to place no value at all on truth telling. When one person spoke to another, there would be no presumption at all that he was telling the truth—for he could just as easily be speaking falsely. Within that society, there would be no reason to pay attention to what anyone says. (I ask you what time it is, and you say "four o'clock." But there is no presumption that you are speaking truly; you could just as easily have said the first thing that came into your head. So I have no reason to pay attention to your answer—in fact, there was no point in my asking you in the first place!) Communication would then be extremely difficult, if not impossible. And because complex societies cannot exist without regular communication among their members, society would become impossible. It follows that in any complex society there must be a presumption in favor of truthfulness. There may of course be exceptions to this rule: there may be situations in which it is thought to be permissible to lie. Nevertheless, these will be exceptions to a rule that is in force in the society. (32)

The prohibition against murder is given as another example of a rule needed for a society to survive. (30) One philosopher has developed the following list of core moral principles binding on all human beings:

1. It is morally wrong to torture people for the fun of it.
2. Do not kill innocent people.
3. Do not cause pain or suffering except when a higher duty prescribes it.
4. Do not commit rape.
5. Keep your promises and contracts.
6. Do not deprive another person of his or her freedom.
7. Do justice, treating equals equally and unequals unequally.
8. Tell the truth.
9. Help other people.
10. Obey just laws. (31)

Among these allegedly common moral principles, [2], [3], [5], [7] and [8] have definite implications for the field of health care.

NOTES

1. Tom L. Beauchamp & James F. Childress, *Principles of Biomedical Ethics*, 5th ed. (New York: Oxford, 2001).
2. Judith Wilson Ross, John W. Glaser, Dorothy Rasinski-Gregory, Joan McIver Gibson, & Corrine Bayley, *Health Care Ethics Committees The Next Generation* (Chicago: American Hospital Publishing, 1993).
3. For a classic description of American individualism, see Robert N. Bellah, Richard Madsen, Willian M. Sullivan, Ann Swidler, & Steven M. Tipton, *Habits of the Heart* (New York: Harper & Row, 1985).
4. Council on Ethical and Judicial Affairs of the American Medical Association,

"Guidelines for the Appropriate Use of Do-Not-Resuscitate Orders," *Journal of the American Medical Association* 265/14 (April 10, 1991): 1868-71.

5. Celia Wolf-Devine, "Abortion and the 'Feminine Voice,' " *Public Affairs Quarterly* 3/3 (July 1989).

6. Tom L. Beauchamp and Leroy Walters (eds.), *Contemporary Issues in Bioethics*, 5th ed. (Belmont, CA: Wadsworth, 1999).

7. Russell E. Smith (ed.), *Conserving Human Life* (Braintree, MA: Pope John Center, 1989).

8. President's Commission for the Study of Ethical Problems in Medicine and Biomedical and Behavioral Research, *Deciding to Forego Life-Sustaining Treatment* (1983; reprint New York: Concern for Dying).

9. Vatican Congregation for the Doctrine of the Faith, *Declaration on Euthanasia* (Washington, DC: United States Catholic Conference, 1980).

10. National Conference of Catholic Bishops, *Ethical and Religious Directives for Catholic Health Care Services* November 1994 (Washington, DC: United States Catholic Conference, 1995).

11. Hastings Center, *Guidelines on the Termination of Life-Sustaining Treatment and the Care of the Dying* (Briarcliff Manor, NY: Hastings Center, 1987).

12. D.J. O'Connor, *Aquinas and Natural Law* (London: Macmillan, 1967).

13. Thomas Hobbes, *Leviathan* (New York: E.P. Dutton, 1950).

14. John Locke, *Essays on the Law of Nature*, trans. W. von Leyden (Oxford: Clarendon, 1965).

15. Vatican Congregation for the Doctrine of the Faith, *Instruction on Respect for Human Life in its Origin and On The Dignity of Procreation* (Washington, DC: United States Catholic Conference, 1987).

16. James F. Gustafson, *Protestant and Roman Catholic Ethics Prospects for Rapprochement* (Chicago: University of Chicago Press, 1978).

17. Orville N. Griese, *Catholic Identity in Health Care: Principles and Practice* (Braintree, MA: Pope John Center, 1987).

18. "Reproductive Control" in Ronald Munson (ed.), *Intervention and Reflection Basic Issues in Medical Ethics*, 5th ed. (Belmont, CA: Wadsworth, 1996).

19. Heidi Malm, "Paid Surrogacy: Arguments and Responses," *Public Affairs Quarterly* 3/2 (April 1989).

20. Elizabeth S. Anderson, "Is Women's Labor a Commodity?" *Philosophy and Public Affairs* 19/1 (Winter 1990).

21. "Utilitarianism" in Ronald Munson (ed.), *Intervention and Reflection Basic Issues in Medical Ethics*, 5th ed. (Belmont, CA: Wadsworth, 1996).

22. Jonathan Harrison, "Utilitarianism, Universalization, and Our Duty to Be Just," *Proceedings of the Aristotelian Society* 53 (1952-3): 105-34.

23. Jeremy Bentham, *An Introduction to the Principles of Morals and Legislation in The Utilitarians* (Garden City, NY: Anchor/Doubleday, 1973).

24. John Stuart Mill, *Utilitarianism* (Indianapolis: Bobbs-Merrill, 1957).

25. "Ethical Theories: Paternalism, Truth Telling, Confidentiality" in Ronald Munson (ed.), *Intervention and Reflection Basic Issues in Medical Ethics*, 5th ed. (Belmont, CA: Wadsworth, 1996).

26. Martin Curd, *Argument and Analysis An Introduction to Philosophy* (St. Paul: West, 1992).

27. Immanuel Kant, *The Foundations of the Metaphysics of Morals*, trans. T.K. Abbott in William H. Shaw (ed.), *Social and Personal Ethics*, 2nd ed. (Belmont, CA: Wadsworth, 1996).

28. "Kant's Ethics" in William H. Shaw (ed.), *Social and Personal Ethics*, 2nd ed. (Belmont, CA: Wadsworth, 1996).

29. Ruth Macklin, "Is There Anything Wrong with Surrogate Motherhood? An Ethical Analysis," *Law, Medicine & Health Care* 16 (1988): 57-64.

30. Case adapted from the video *Human Experiments: The Price of Knowledge?* (KCTS/Seattle, 1980).

31. Louis Pojman, "Ethical Relativism versus Ethical Objectivism" in Louis P. Pojman, *Introduction to Philosophy Classical and Contemporary Readings* (Belmont, CA: Wadsworth, 1991).

32. James Rachels, "The Challenge of Cultural Relativism" in Joel Feinberg, *Reason and Responsibility Readings in Some Basic Problems of Philosophy*, 9th ed. (Belmont, CA: Wadsworth, 1996).

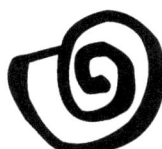

Index

www.ingramcontent.com/pod-product-compliance
Lightning Source LLC
Chambersburg PA
CBHW061357210326
41598CB00035B/6018